T0093469

Phytochemistry of
Withania somnifera

Phytochemical Investigations of Medicinal Plants

Series Editor: Brijesh Kumar

Phytochemistry of Plants of Genus Phyllanthus
Brijesh Kumar, Sunil Kumar and K.P. Madhusudanan

Phytochemistry of Plants of Genus Ocimum
Brijesh Kumar, Vikas Bajpai, Surabhi Tiwari and Renu Pandey

Phytochemistry of Plants of Genus Piper
Brijesh Kumar, Surabhi Tiwari, Vikas Bajpai and Bikarma Singh

Phytochemistry of Tinospora cordifolia
Brijesh Kumar, Vikas Bajpai and Nikhil Kumar

Phytochemistry of Plants of Genus Rauvolfia
Brijesh Kumar, Sunil Kumar, Vikas Bajpai and K.P. Madhusudanan

Phytochemistry of Piper betle Landacres
Vikas Bajpai, Nikhil Kumar and Brijesh Kumar

Phytochemical Investigations of Genus Terminalia
Brijesh Kumar, Awantika Singh and K.P. Madhusudanan

Phytochemistry of Plants of Genus Cassia
Brijesh Kumar, Vikas Bajpai, Vikaskumar Gond, Subhashis Pal and Naibedya Chattopadhyay

Phytochemistry of Withania Somnifera
Brijesh Kumar, Vikas Bajpai, Vikaskumar Gond, Surabhi Tiwari and K.P. Madhusudanan

For more information about this series, please visit: https://www.crcpress.com/Phytochemical-Investigations-of-Medicinal-Plants/book-series/PHYTO

Phytochemistry of
Withania somnifera

Brijesh Kumar, Vikas Bajpai,
Vikaskumar Gond, Surabhi Tiwari
and K.P. Madhusudanan

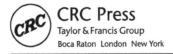

CRC Press
Taylor & Francis Group
Boca Raton London New York

CRC Press is an imprint of the
Taylor & Francis Group, an **informa** business

First edition published 2022
by CRC Press
6000 Broken Sound Parkway NW, Suite 300, Boca Raton, FL 33487-2742
and by CRC Press

4 Park Square, Milton Park, Abingdon, Oxon, OX14 4RN

CRC Press is an imprint of Taylor & Francis Group, LLC

ISBN: 978-1-032-03019-7 (hbk)
ISBN: 978-1-032-03020-3 (pbk)
ISBN: 978-1-003-18627-4 (ebk)

DOI: 10.1201/9781003186274

Typeset in Times
by KnowledgeWorks Global Ltd.

Contents

List of Figures

List of Tables

Preface

Plants are considered as one of the most important sources of modern medicine. They have been used for different ailments of human beings worldwide since the beginning of civilization. Bioactive secondary metabolites have been considered as a fundamental source of medicine for the treatment of a range of diseases in the modern medical system. India has a rich heritage of medicinal plants which are the basis of indigenous systems of medicine such as Ayurveda, Siddha, Unani, Homoeopathy and Naturopathy. In India, about 6000–7000 plant species are utilized in traditional, folk and herbal medicine. Herbal medicines/formulations involve the use of crude or processed plants containing several active constituents. Identification and determination of the active constituents are the crucial prerequisites for the development of modern evidence-based phytomedicine. The use of medicinal herbs or herbal drugs is increasing throughout the world, though one of the main encumbrances in its acceptance globally is the lack of quality control or standardization. Standardization is an essential step for the establishment of consistent pharmacological activity. A reliable chemical profile or simply, a quality control program for the production of herbal drugs from medicinal plants can serve the purpose. Herbal medicines have good potential in treating many diseases including noninfectious diseases like cancer and diabetes. Recently, interest in traditional medicines in India has been increasing due to the belief that these are much safer, nontoxic in nature and without any side effects. This has been proven in the treatment of various ailments. Phytochemical analysis provides the relationship between the composition of complex and variable mixtures of plant-derived medicines and their biological effects.

Withania somnifera, commonly known as Ashwagandha, is a plant used in medicine from the time of Ayurveda, the ancient system of Indian medicine. In the traditional system of Indian medicine, it is used as a tonic to rejuvenate the body and increase longevity. In Ayurvedic preparations, various parts of the plant have been used to treat a variety of ailments that affect the human health. It showed antioxidant, abortifacient, antibiotic, aphrodisiac, deobstruent, diuretic, sedative, antidiabetic, immunomodulatory, hemopoietic, and neuroprotective properties. Its chemo-preventive properties make it a potentially useful adjunct for patients receiving radiation and chemotherapy. This book describes the quantitative analysis of phytochemicals in

W. somnifera by liquid chromatography mass spectrometric methods. UPLC-ESI-QqQLIT MS/MS methods were found to be effective for quantitation of phytochemicals in different varieties of *W. somnifera* grown in different soil conditions. This method is also applicable to control the quality of commercial herbal formulations containing *W. somnifera*. Herbal analysis is a thrust area and an essential requirement to improve the traditional knowledge of herbal medicines. It describes the use of statistical softwares (PCA, HCA, Factor analysis, etc.) in phytochemical determinations in different varieties of the plant. Markers were identified for quality control and authentication.

Acknowledgements

The completion of this book is due to the Almighty, who blessed us with all the resources required to accomplish this journey. We are glad to have this chance to express our gratitude to people who have been supportive to us at every time. We are also thankful to Dr. Preeti Chandra for her constant support on this book. We express our deep sense of gratitude to the Director, CSIR-Central Drug Research Institute (CDRI), Lucknow for his support and Sophisticated Analytical Instrument Facility (SAIF) Division, CSIR-CDRI, India where all the data were generated.

Authors

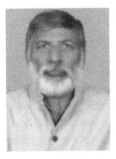

Brijesh Kumar, PhD, was a Professor (AcSIR) and Chief Scientist at sophisticated analytical instrument facility division, CSIR-Central Drug Research Institute, Lucknow, India. He earned a PhD at CSIR-CDRI, Lucknow (Dr. Ram Manohar Lohia, Avadh University Faizabad UP, India). He has written eight books, 11 book chapters and 151 papers in reputed international journals. His area of research is applications of mass spectrometry for qualitative and quantitative analysis of Indian medicinal plants and their herbal formulations for quality control and authentication/standardization. He is also involved in the identification of marker compounds using statistical software to check adulteration/substitution.

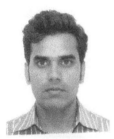

Vikas Bajpai, PhD, earned a PhD at the Academy of Scientific and Innovative Research (AcSIR), New Delhi, India, and conducted research work under the supervision of Dr. Brijesh Kumar at CSIR-Central Drug Research Institute Lucknow. His research includes the development and validation of LC-MS/MS methods for qualitative and quantitative analysis of small molecules of Indian medicinal plants.

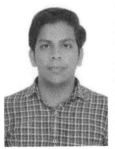

Vikaskumar Gond is a junior research fellow working under the supervision of Dr. Brijesh Kumar in the mass spectrometry laboratory, Sophisticated Analytical Instrument Facility at CSIR-Central Drug Research Institute, Lucknow. He earned a master's in pharmaceutical chemistry at the University of Lucknow. His research interests include the finger-printing and characterization of phytochemicals using LC-MS/MS.

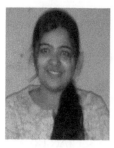

Surabhi Tiwari earned a master's in chemistry at the University of Allahabad, India. After working on the analysis of herbals using instruments such as HPTLC and HPLC in the Pharmacognosy Division, NBRI, Lucknow, she is a Senior Research Fellow in the SAIF Division of CSIR-Central Drug Research Institute, Lucknow, India, under the supervision of Dr. Brijesh Kumar. Her research interests include the phytochemical analysis of medicinal plants.

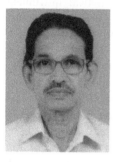

K.P. Madhusudanan, PhD, is a mass spectrometry scientist. He earned a PhD in organic mass spectrometry at the National Chemical Laboratory, Pune, India. He worked as a scientist and head, Sophisticated Analytical Instrument Facility in Central Drug Research Institute, Lucknow until 2007. His research includes various aspects of organic mass spectrometry, such as fragmentation mechanism, gas phase unusual reactions, positive and negative ion mass spectrometry of natural products using various ionization techniques including DART, effects of metal cationization, LC/MS and MS/MS applications and quantitative analysis of drugs and metabolites. He has written more than 150 research publications. He was a member of the editorial board of *Journal of Mass Spectrometry* from 1995 to 2007. He is a fellow of the National Academy of Sciences, Allahabad, India.

List of Abbreviations and Units

°C	degree Celsius
μg	microgram
μL	microlitre
APCI	atmospheric pressure chemical ionization
API	atmospheric pressure ionization
BPC	base peak chromatogram
CAD	collision-activated dissociation
CE	capillary electrophoresis
CE	collision energy
CEC	cation-exchange capacity
CID	collision-induced dissociation
CXP	cell exit potential
Da	Dalton
DAD	diode array detection
DP	declustering potential
DTPA	diethylenetriaminepentaacetic acid
EC	electrical conductivity
EP	entrance potential
ESI	electrospray ionization
ESP	exchangeable sodium percent
FDA	Food and Drug Administration
FIA	flow injection analysis
g	gram
GC-MS	gas chromatography-mass spectrometry
GS1	nebulizer gas
GS2	heater gas
h	hour
HCA	hierarchical clustering analysis
HPLC	high performance liquid chromatography
HR-MAS	high resolution magic angle spinning
ICH	International Conference on Harmonization

IS	internal standard
IT	ion trap
kPa	kilopascal
L	litre
LC	liquid chromatography
LOD	limit of detection
LOQ	limit of quantification
LTQ	linear trap quadrupole
MALDI TOF MS	matrix-assisted laser desorption ionization time of flight mass spectrometry
m/z	mass to charge ratio
mg	milligram
min	minute
mL	millilitre
mM	millimolar
MRM	multiple reaction monitoring
MS	mass spectrometry
ms	millisecond
MS/MS	tandem mass spectrometry
ng	nanogram
NMR	nuclear magnetic resonance
PCA	principal component analysis
PDA	photodiode array detection
psi	pressure per square inch
QqQ$_{LIT}$	hybrid linear ion trap triplequadrupole
QTOF	quadrupole time of flight
r^2	correlation coefficient
RDA	retro-Diels-Alder
RSD	relative standard deviation
S/N	signal to noise ratio
SD	standard deviation
t$_R$	retention time
UPLC	ultra performance liquid chromatography
UPLC-QqQ$_{LIT}$-MS/MS	ultra high performance liquid chromatography hybrid linear ion trap triplequadrupole tandem mass spectrometry
UV	ultraviolet
WHO	World Health Organization
W. somnifera	*Withinia somnifera*
WS	*Withinia somnifera*
XIC/EIC	extracted ion chromatogram

Withania
Ethno and Phytopharmacological Review

1

1.1 INTRODUCTION

Plants have been used in folk and traditional medicines for thousands of years (Petrovska 2012). One of the oldest, richest and most diverse cultural traditions of use of medicinal plants for human health is in India. The earliest records of treatment with plants can be found in the holy books of Vedas. Ayurveda (the science of life), the Indian system of traditional medicine, traces its roots to Atharvaveda and is known to have developed from the knowledge accumulated for centuries. About 10,000 plants are used for medicinal purposes in the Indian subcontinent. But only 1200–1500 plants are part of the Ayurvedic Pharmacopeia in more than 3000 years (Kumar et al. 2017). This clearly shows that Ayurveda investigates the plants well before including them as Ayurvedic medicine (Manohar 2012). *Withania somnifera* (L.) Dunal from Solanaceae (nightshade or potato) family, commonly known in India as Ashwagandha, is an important medicinal plant widely used in Ayurveda and other indigenous systems of medicine for over 3000 years (Patwardhan et al. 1988; Tuli and Sangwan 2009). Ashwagandha has been used since ancient times to relieve stress, increase energy levels and improve concentration, to lower blood sugar and cortisol levels and to treat anxiety and depression (Rege et al. 1999; Winters 2006; Mirjalili et al. 2009a). It is also known as winter cherry, poison gooseberry or Indian ginseng. The Sanskrit

DOI: 10.1201/9781003186274-1

name 'ashwagandha' roughly translates to the 'smell and strength of a horse' hinting at its traditional use to enhance sex drive. The root has a strong horse-like aroma. The genus *Withania* is named after Henry Witham, an English paleobotanist of the early 19th century (Purdie et al. 1982). The species name *somnifera* (Latin, meaning 'sleep-inducing') is justified by its use to support somnolence. 'Dunal' is used to honour the French botanist Michel Felix Dunal (1789–1856) involved in classifying Solanaceous plant genus. Ashwagandha is used in India as a general tonic effective against a large number of ailments similar to how ginseng is used in traditional Chinese medicine to treat a large variety of human diseases and hence it is also referred to as Indian ginseng (Kulkarni and Dhir 2008).

It is known by different names in other languages: asgandh or ajagandha in Hindi, asbagandha in Bengali, amukkara in Tamil, amukkuram in Malayalam, askandha in Marathi, asod in Gujarati and so on. Ashwagandha is a foundational and cure-all herb in Ayurveda, wherein it is classified as 'Rasayana' (tonic) capable of rejuvenating the body, enhancing haemoglobin count and hair melanin pigmentation, memory, physiological endurance and general health, promoting defense against diseases and arresting the ageing process (Singh et al. 2011a). In Ayurveda, its clinical uses include treatment of general debility, emaciation, consumption, constipation, nervous exhaustion, impotence, insomnia, loss of memory and premature ageing (Warrier et al. 1996).

The genus *Withania* is closely related to the genus *Physalis*, the gooseberries. *Physalis somnifera* L., *Withania kansuensis* Kuang & A. M. Lu and *Withania microphysalis* Suess. are synonyms of *W. somnifera*. Dunal (Tropicos 2021). Being a family of trees, shrubs and herbs, the Solanaceae (the nightshade or the potato family) has 95 genera and 3000 species distributed throughout the world. *Withania* is a genus of the nightshade family of flowering plants distributed in the subtropical regions from the Mediterranean to South East Asia. Only two species *W. somnifera* and *W. coagulans* are found in India (Chadha 1976). The most common species is *W. somnifera* (WS) occurring naturally in the subtropical regions from the Mediterranean through Africa to the Middle East, Indian continent, Sri Lanka, South East Asia, subtropical America and Australia (Kulkarni and Dhir 2008). WS is a native to the drier parts of India up to an altitude of 1500 m. It is also largely cultivated, on a commercial scale, in the states of Punjab, Rajasthan, Haryana, Uttar Pradesh, Gujarat, Maharashtra, Madhya Pradesh and Karnataka and also in other parts of the world, mainly for its fleshy roots (Goraya and Ved 2017; Srivastava et al. 2018). It is a perennial shrub that grows to 75 cm in height with tomentose branches, oval yellowish green leaves, orange red berries and a papery calyx and it survives harsh climatic conditions. In Ayurveda, it is believed that the plants which survive harsh conditions have strong healing and tonification properties (Forman and Kerna 2018).

1.2 TRADITIONAL USES AND MEDICINAL PROPERTIES

Ethnopharmacology, traditional uses and phytoconstituents of WS have been reviewed recently (Mukherjee et al. 2021). WS can be easily recognized by its orange, red fruit covered with brownish, inflated calyx and its leaves having a strong smell of green tomatoes and strong-smelling (horse-like) roots which are stout, fleshy and whitish brown. The fruit is relished by birds. The roots, leaves and berries possess medicinal values and hence used in many tonics and formulations as a rejuvenative botanical to nourish muscles and bones, while enhancing the function of the adrenals and reproductive system (Umadevi et al. 2012). WS is an ancient plant with remarkable therapeutic uses in both traditional and modern medicine. WS in Ayurvedic medicine is similar to ginseng in traditional Chinese medicine. It is one of the best health tonics and restorative medicines useful to treat general debility. It is used as a 'Rasayana' which promotes a youthful state of physical and mental health as a promoter of strength, learning and memory, longevity and sexual health, arresting the ageing process, revitalizing the body in debilitated conditions and improving defense against diseases. WS is traditionally used as a rejuvenative tonic to relieve general debility during convalescence or old age, a sleep inducer, a sedative and a nervine tonic for memory enhancement (Singh et al. 2011a). Therapeutic properties and significance of different parts of WS are summarized (Pratibha et al. 2013).

Among the plant parts of WS, the root is the most medicinally useful. It is bitter, anthelmintic, deobstruent, narcotic, astringent, thermogenic, aphrodisiac, germicidal, restorative and diuretic. It cures ulcers, fever, dropsy, impotence, rheumatism and leucoderma. It is a tonic that improves physical strength and hence used in general debility. The root boosts the immune system and increases the white cell count and regulates blood sugar levels, and reduces bad cholesterol level. It has mild sedative properties that promote sound sleep. According to folklore, its root is used for cold, fever, asthma, tuberculosis and as an abortifacient. The roots are also used for treating constipation, nervous breakdown, goitre, joint inflammation (Singh et al. 2011a), ulcers and painful swellings (Kirtikar and Basu 1935), pimples, worms, piles, leucorrhoea and pulmonary tuberculosis (Mishra 2004). WS root, its powder and paste are used for rheumatic pain, arthritis, cardiopulmonary disorder, constipation, loss of memory, abortion, inflammation of joints, nervous disorder, epilepsy, glandular swelling, ulcers, female sterility, digestive disorders, rheumatic arthritis, general debility, insomnia and tumors (Puri 2002; Datta et al. 2011). It is a sex tonic that helps to cure erectile dysfunction and spermatorrhea. It also tones up the uterus of women. It is anti-inflammatory and helps to relieve back pain and sciatica. The root powder can be consumed with milk or honey. A paste of the root/leaf powder helps to cure carbuncles and swellings. It is also used as an aphrodisiac, diuretic, restorative and rejuvenative. The roots and leaves boost cognition, relieve gastrointestinal ailments, correct thyroid dysfunction, counter stress and promote immunity and general health (Rege et al. 1999). The crushed leaves are applied externally for joint pains, inflammation and boils (Datta et al. 2011). Traditionally, WS is taken in its powdered form mixed with honey or ghee. It can also be taken as a tea with milk. The root in combination with other drugs is prescribed for scorpion sting and snake bite. In rural India, WS is applied externally as an antidote for snake bite.

The leaves of this plant are bitter, anthelmintic and anti-inflammatory, and are used to treat fever, syphilis, hemorrhoids and painful swellings. It is also used to treat sore eyes, boils and swollen hands and feet by fomentation. Paste of the leaves is used to eradicate body lice and also useful for carbuncles, bed sore, wounds, ulcers, skin infections and swelling. A paste made from the fresh leaves and roots is applied externally to boils, swelling and rheumatism (Quattrocchi 2012). The leaves can also be consumed by making its tea. The leaves are aphrodisiac, diuretic and narcotic (Puri 2002). The flowers are astringent, aphrodisiac and diuretic and are considered purifying and detoxifying (Singh et al. 2011a). The fruits are anthelmintic, emetic and stomachic, blood purifier and febrifuge, sedative, alternative, diuretic and bitter tonic in dyspepsia as well as a growth promoter in infants (Singh and Kumar 1998). It is also used for the treatment of asthma, atherosclerosis, intestinal and liver disorders (Thakur et al. 1989). The fruits are used to treat wounds, ulcers and tubercular glands. The berries and seeds are anthelmintic, diuretic, narcotic and hypnotic (Singh et al. 2011a). The berries are used as a substitute for rennet, to coagulate milk in cheese making and this property is attributed to the pulp and the husk of the berry (Facciola 1990) The fruits and seeds are rich in saponins and can be used as a substitute for soap (Saritha and Naidu 2007).

WS is primarily used as a fine powder called 'Churna' which easily mixes with water, milk, honey or other fluids. The common method of traditional 'rasayana' preparation is boiling the herb directly in milk, as milk is thought to leach out undesirable constituents and augment the tonifying and nutritive effects. At present, people prefer taking WS as a powder in capsule form (Frawley and Lad 2016). It is an ancient herb, giving modern benefits. It is one of the ingredients in more than 100 Ayurvedic herbal formulations (Singh and Kumar 1998). The traditional uses of WS can be summarized as follows: it combats stress, helps to calm down, boosts stamina, stimulates endocrine system and restores body balance leading to rejuvenation. It fights depression, enhances mood, reduces swelling and pain, boosts memory and cognitive performance and prevents cancer cell growth. It has the remarkable ability to induce restful sleep and improve sexual health in man and woman. It is prescribed in case of debility to promote strength, vigour and vitality and acts as an adaptogen fortifying the immune system. After thousands of years of continuous use, WS is still regarded as one of the most valuable medicinal herbs and an ancient medicine in modern times (Samadi 2013).

1.3 PHYTOCHEMICAL CONSTITUENTS

The main bioactive phytoconstituents of WS are withasteroids or withanolides, alkaloids, flavonoids, sterols, phenolics and others. Withanolides are a group of naturally occurring C_{28}-steroidal lactones built on an intact or rearranged ergostane framework (Ray and Gupta 1994). Among the various withanolides, withanolide A, withaferin A, withanone and withanolide D are the most abundant having various activities (Sangwan et al. 2017). Other abundant phytochemicals include withanamides (A, B, C, D, E), withanosides, withanolide glycosides, steroidal saponins, lignanamides, flavonoids, coagulins, tropane alkaloids (calistegins, pseudotropine and tropine), fatty acids, organic acids, amino acids, sugars and sterol-based compounds distributed among different plant parts (Mirjalili et al. 2009a, Chatterjee et al. 2010; Sangwan et al. 2017). The distribution of secondary metabolites varies with the nature of the tissues (leaf, root, stem, fruit), stage of development and chemotypes (Chatterjee et al. 2010; Dhar et al. 2013). It has been shown that leaves as compared to roots constitute the main tissue for accumulation of withanolides (Dhar et al. 2013).

The major metabolites present in leaves are withaferin A and withanone, whereas withanolide A and withanolide D are the major metabolites present in roots (Singh et al. 2015a). The earthy odour and flavour of WS is attributed to the presence of steroidal lactones or withanolides. Phytochemical and pharmacological activities have been reviewed by several workers (Gupta and Rana 2007). Another review summarized the withanolides reported during 1996–2009 and their pharmacological activities (Singh et al. 2010a). There are several other reviews on withanolides (Ray and Gupta 1994; Misico et al. 2011; Choudhary et al. 2013). According to a review in 2009, the phytoconstituents of WS isolated and reported from aerial parts, roots and berries include more than 12 alkaloids, 40 withanolides and several sitoindosides (Mirjalili et al. 2009a). Chen et al. (2011) provided a comprehensive summary of the 360 naturally occurring withanolides isolated and identified during 1996–2010 from plants of the Nightshade family. Withaferin A was discovered in 1965 from WS and since then up to 2014 exhaustive research has resulted in the discovery of 167 natural products including 127 C_{28}-ergostane steroids (withanolides),

19 alkaloids, five withanolide precursors, four flavonoids, three phenolic acids, two coumarins and five miscellaneous compounds (Zhang and Timmermann 2014). Chemical constituents of pharmacological importance identified in various parts of WS are listed in a recent report (Rayees and Malik 2017). Phytochemical composition, medicinal applications and nutrapharmaceutical potentials of WS have been reviewed recently (Saleem et al. 2020). The structural, biological and pharmacological activities of more than 170 new withanolides isolated and identified in the last 5 years are summarized in a recent review (Xu and Wang 2020). The phytochemical constituents (138) reported in leaves, roots and aerial parts of WS and detected by thin layer chromatography (TLC), high performance thin layer chromatography (HPTLC), high performance liquid chromatography (HPLC), electrospray ionization-mass spectrometry (ESI-MS), gas chromatography-mass spectrometry (GC-MS), liquid chromatography-mass spectrometry (LC-MS) or nuclear magnetic resonance (NMR) are listed by Tetali et al. (2021).

Withasomnine, anaferine, tropine, pseudotropine, anahygrine and somniferine (1-(3-4-dimethoxybenzyl)-6-7-dimethoxyisoquinoline) were found to be the predominant alkaloids in the roots of WS (Sharma et al. 2013). The steroidal withanolides of WS resemble the ginsenosides found in *Panax ginseng* (Ginseng) both in structure and activity (Singh et al. 2011a). Withanolides are mainly localized in leaves and roots, although they have been reported from all the plant parts (Sangwan et al. 2008). The concentration of major withanolides ranges from 0.001 to 0.5% on dry weight basis (Atal et al. 1975; Kapur 2001). Their concentrations depend on factors, such as cultivar, age of the plant, growth rate, geographical location, soil and environmental conditions (Vaishnavi et al. 2013). The most abundant withanolide in WS is withaferin A (Chaurasiya et al. 2008; Misra et al. 2008). Its presence in leaves is 27 times more than that in the roots (Gajbhiye et al. 2015). There are several other reviews discussing the phytochemical constituents of WS (Gavande et al. 2015; Kumar et al. 2015a; Kalra and Kaushik 2017). A few more withanolides and other constituents have been identified recently. Mahrous et al. (2019) isolated two withanolides, withaperuvin C, phyperunolide F, a lipid 1,2-di-O-palmitoyl-3-O-(6‴-sulfo-α-D-quinovopyranosyl)-glycerol and β-sitosterol glucoside from Egyptian WS leaf extract and two lipids, 1,3-dicaproyl-2-vaccenoyl glycerol, vaccenoyl monoglyceride and a fatty acid vaccenic acid from the ripe fruit extract. Mahrous et al. (2017) had earlier isolated withanolide S from Egyptian *Withania*. Six new cytotoxic withanolides, withasilolides A–F were identified and characterized by spectroscopic methods in MeOH extract of WS roots (Kim et al. 2019). Several alkaloids (Filipiak-Szok et al. 2017), flavonoids (Mundkinajeddu et al. 2014; Filipiak-Szok et al. 2017; Hameed and Akhtar 2018; Funde 2019; El-Hefny et al. 2020), phenolics and phenolic acids (Singh et al. 2016; Filipiak-Szok et al. 2017; Hameed and Akhtar 2018; El-Hefny et al. 2020) and phenyl propanoid esters (Baek et al. 2019) have also been identified recently. Trivedi et al. (2017) identified dihydrowithanolide D and ixocarpalactone A in the hydroalcoholic root extract of WS along with other known withanolides (a total of 43 possible withanolides) based on liquid chromatography-electrospray ionization mass spectrometry (LC-ESIMS), GC-MS and NMR studies. Fatty acids such as palmitic, oleic, linoleic and linolenic acids have been isolated from *n*-hexane extracts of the leaves and roots of WS (Chatterjee et al. 2010).

Metabolic profiling of the hexane extracts of WS fruits using GC-MS and aqueous methanolic extracts using ^{1}H NMR revealed 82 chemically diverse metabolites including organic acids, fatty acids, aliphatic and aromatic amino acids, polyols, sugars and sugar alcohols, sterols, tocopherols, phenolic acids and withanamides (Bhatia et al. 2013). Out of 82 constituents, 32 were volatile and detected in GC-MS, whereas the remaining were polar constituents detected using ^{1}H NMR spectroscopy. Squalene and tocopherol have been identified for the first time in the fruits of WS. Cycloartenol (a precursor to phytosterols), cholesterol, campesterol, sitosterol and stigmasterol were also detected (Bhatia et al. 2013). In a recent study on the determination of selected alkaloids, flavonoids and phenolic acids in WS, the predominant alkaloids, though in much lower concentration than flavonoids and phenolic acids, were found to be caffeine, harman and berberine (Filipiak-Szok et al. 2017). Flavonoids quercetin and rutin were the predominant flavonols. Gallic acid was the most abundant phenolic acid (Filipiak-Szok et al. 2017). The major phytoconstituents of WS identified and characterized are given in Table 1.1.

1.4 PHARMACOLOGICAL AND CLINICAL RESEARCH

1.4.1 Major Activities

WS is a wonder herb with a broad spectrum of pharmacological properties such as antioxidant, antidepressant, aphrodisiac, antiulcerogenic, antivenom, anti-inflammatory, antiarthritic, anticancer, antiparasitic, antimicrobial, anticancerous, antidiabetic, antitumor, hemopoietic neuroregenerative, immunomodulatory, cardioprotective, radiosensitizing, rejuvinating, antistress, sedative, hypoglycemic, thyroprotective, adaptogenic, antispasmodic, immunomodulatory, immunostimulant and antiageing properties (Vyas et al. 2011; Mir et al. 2012; Uddin et al. 2012; Patel et al. 2013; Dar et al. 2015; Halder and

TABLE 1.1 Phytochemicals reported in *W. somnifera*

COMPOUND	PLANT PART	REFERENCE
Withanolides (Partial list)		
Ashwagandhanolide	Root	Subbaraju et al. 2006
Coagulin Q	Root	Zhao et al. 2002
27-Deoxy withaferin A	Leaves	Zhang and Timmermann 2014
12-Deoxy withastramonolide	Plant materials	Penman et al. 2007
Dihydrowithanolide D	Root	Trivedi et al. 2017
6α, 7α-Epoxy-5α, 14α, 17α, 23β-tetrahydroxy-1-oxo-22R-witha-2, 24-dienolide	Fruits	Abou-Douh 2002
6α,7α-Epoxy-1α, 3β, 5α-trihydroxy-witha-24-enolide	Berries	Lal et al. 2006
27-Hydroxy withanolide A	Roots, berries	Zhang and Timmermann 2014
27-Hydroxy withanolide B	Leaves, roots	Zhang and Timmermann 2014
27-Hydroxy withanone	Leaves	Misra et al. 2005
Iso-withanone	Berries	Lal et al. 2006
Ixocarpalactone A	Root	Trivedi et al. 2017
5β, 6α, 14α, 17β, 20β-Pentahydroxy-1-oxo-20 S, 22R-witha-2, 24-dienolide	Fruits	Abou-Douh 2002
Phyperunolide F	Leaves	Mahrous et al. 2019
Physagulin D	Leaves	Jayaprakasam and Nair 2003
Sitoindoside VII	Roots	Bhattacharya et al. 1987
Sitoindoside VIII	Roots	Bhattacharya et al. 1987
Sitoindoside IX	Roots	Ghosal et al. 1989
Sitoindoside X	Roots, leaves, aerial parts	Ghosal et al. 1989
Withaferin A	Leaves, whole plants, aerial parts, roots	Lavie et al. 1965; Zhang and Timmermann 2014
Withanolide A-Z	Roots/leaves	Zhang and Timmermann 2014
Withanone	Leaves, berries, roots	Dhalla et al. 1961; Lal et al. 2006; Ismail 2013
Withanoside I-XI	Roots/fruits/leaves	Matsuda et al. 2001; Zhao et al. 2002

(Continued)

TABLE 1.1 (Continued) Phytochemicals reported in *W. somnifera*

COMPOUND	PLANT PART	REFERENCE
Withaperuvin C	Leaves	Mahrous et al. 2019
Withasilolides A-F	Roots	Kim et al. 2019
Alkaloids		
Anaferine	Roots	Schwarting et al. 1963; Sharma et al. 2013
Anahygrine	Roots	Schwarting et al. 1963; Sharma et al. 2013
Berberine	Roots	Filipiak-Szok et al. 2017
Caffeine	Fruits/roots	El-Hefny et al. 2020; Filipiak-Szok et al. 2017
Choline	Roots/leaves	Schwarting et al. 1963; Chatterjee et al. 2010
Cuscohygrine	Roots	Schwarting et al. 1963; Sharma et al. 2013
Harmane	Roots	Filipiak-Szok et al. 2017
Harmine	Roots	Filipiak-Szok et al. 2017
Isopelletierine	Roots	Schwarting et al. 1963; Sharma et al. 2013
Nicotine	Roots	Majumdar 1955
Noscapine	Roots	Filipiak-Szok et al. 2017
Papaverine	Roots	Filipiak-Szok et al. 2017
Pseudo-tropine	Roots	Schwarting et al. 1963; Sharma et al. 2013
(+)-Sedridine	Root	Sonar et al. 2015
Somniferine [1-(3-4—dimethoxybenzyl)-6-7-dimethoxyiso-quinoline]	Roots	Sharma et al. 2013
Theobromine	Roots	Filipiak-Szok et al. 2017
Theophylline	Roots	Filipiak-Szok et al. 2017
3α-Tigloyloxytropane	Roots	Schwarting et al. 1963
Tropine	Roots	Schwarting et al. 1963
Withanamides A-I	Fruits	Jayaprakasam et al. 2004
Withasomnine	Roots	Schröter et al. 1966; Sharma et al. 2013
Yohimbine	Roots	Filipiak-Szok et al. 2017

(Continued)

TABLE 1.1 (Continued)   Phytochemicals reported in *W. somnifera*

COMPOUND	PLANT PART	REFERENCE
Flavonoids		
Apigenin	Berries	Hameed and Akhtar 2018
Catechin	Fruits, leaves, roots, berries	Alam et al. 2011; Hameed and Akhtar 2018
6,8-Dihydroxykaempferol 3-rutinoside	Leaves	Kandil et al. 1994
Hyperoside	Roots	Filipiak-Szok et al. 2017
Kaempferol	Berries/Fruits/root	Hameed and Akhtar 2018; El-Hefny et al. 2020; Filipiak-Szok et al. 2017; Alam et al. 2011
Kaempferol 3-*O*-robinobioside-7-*O*-glucoside	Aerial parts	Mundkinajeddu et al. 2014
Myricetin	Roots/fruits/berries	Filipiak-Szok et al. 2017; El-Hefny et al. 2020; Hameed and Akhtar 2018
Naringenin	Whole plant/fruits	Funde 2019; Alam et al. 2011
Naringin	Whole plant	Funde 2019
Quercetin	Roots/leaves/whole plant	Filipiak-Szok et al. 2017; Kandil et al. 1994; Funde 2019
Quercetin -3-O-galactosyl	Leaves	Bashir et al. 2013
Quercetin 3-*O*-robinobioside-7-*O*-glucoside	Aerial parts	Mundkinajeddu et al. 2014
Quercetin-3-rutinoside-7-glucoside	Leaves, aerial parts	Kandil et al. 1994; Mundkinajeddu et al. 2014
Quercitrin	Roots	Filipiak-Szok et al. 2017
Rhamnetin	Roots	Filipiak-Szok et al. 2017
Rutin	Roots /shoots/ fruits/whole plant/ leaves/berries	Nile and Park 2015; El-Hefny et al. 2020; Funde 2019; Filipiak-Szok et al. 2017; Kandil et al. 1994; Hameed and Akhtar 2018
7, 3′, 4′- Trihydroxy flavone-3-O-rhamnosyl	Leaves	Bashir et al. 2013

(Continued)

TABLE 1.1 (Continued) Phytochemicals reported in *W. somnifera*

COMPOUND	PLANT PART	REFERENCE
5, 7, 4'- Trihydroxy-methyl-3-O-galactosyl flavonol	Leaves	Bashir et al. 2013
Phytosterols		
Campesterol	Roots	Chatterjee et al. 2010
Cholesterol	Fruits	Bhatia et al. 2013
Cycloartenol	Fruits	Bhatia et al. 2013
Sitostanone	Roots	Misra et al. 2012
Stigmasterol	Roots/fruits	Misra et al. 2008, 2012; Chatterjee et al. 2010; Abou-Douh 2002
Stigmasterol glucoside	Roots	Misra et al. 2008
Stigmasterone	Root	Misra et al. 2012
β-Sitosterol	Roots/ fruits	Misra et al. 2008; Abou-Douh 2002
β-Sitosterol glucoside	Roots/leaves	Misra et al. 2008; Mahrous et al. 2019
Phenolic acids/Phenols		
Caffeic acid	Fruits, roots, leaves	El-Hefny et al. 2020; Filipiak-Szok et al. 2017; Singh et al. 2016
4-O-Caffeoyl quinic acid	Leaves	Kandil et al. 1994
Chlorogenic acid	Leaves/roots/whole plant	Singh et al. 2016; Filipiak-Szok et al. 2017; Funde 2019
o-Coumaric acid	Leaves	Singh et al. 2016
p-Coumaric acid	Fruits, roots, leaves	El-Hefny et al. 2020; Filipiak-Szok et al.2017; Alam et al. 2011
Curcumin	Whole plant	Funde 2019
4,5-O-Dicaffeoyl quinic acid	Leaves	Kandil et al. 1994
Ellagic acid	Fruits	El-Hefny et al. 2020
Ferulic acid	Fruits, roots, leaves	El-Hefny et al. 2020; Filipiak-Szok et al. 2017; Singh et al. 2016

(Continued)

TABLE 1.1 (Continued)   Phytochemicals reported in *W. somnifera*

COMPOUND	PLANT PART	REFERENCE
Gallic acid	Fruits/ Roots/leaves/ berries/whole plant	El-Hefny et al. 2020; Filipiak-Szok et al. 2017; Singh et al. 2016; Hameed and Akhtar 2018; Alam et al. 2011; Funde 2019
p-Hydroxy benzoic acid	Roots	Filipiak-Szok et al. 2017
2-Hydroxycinnamic acid	Fruits	El-Hefny et al. 2020
p-Hydroxy phenyl acetic acid	Roots	Chatterjee et al. 2010
Phenyl acetic acid	Leaves /roots	Chatterjee et al. 2010
Quinic acid	Leaves	Kandil et al. 1994
Salicylic acid	Fruits/acetone ext	El-Hefny et al. 2020
Syringic acid	Leaves	Alam et al. 2011
3,4,5-Trihydroxy cinnamic acid	Roots	Chatterjee et al. 2010
Vanillic acid	Fruits/leaves	El-Hefny et al. 2020; Alam et al. 2011
Vanillin	Fruits	El-Hefny et al. 2020
Fatty acids & Lipids		
Arachidic acid & others	Fruits	Bhatia et al. 2013
1,3- Dicaproyl-,2-vaccenoyl-glycerol	Fruits	Mahrous et al. 2019
1,2-Di-O-palmitoyl-3-O-(6‴-sulfo-α-D-quinovopyranosyl)-glycerol	Leaves	Mahrous et al. 2019
Hydroxypalmitic acid diglucoside	Fruits	Bolleddula et al. 2012
Linoleic acid	Leaves/roots	Chatterjee et al. 2010
Linolenic acid	Leaves/roots	Chatterjee et al. 2010
Oleic acid	Roots/leaves	Misra et al. 2012; Chatterjee et al. 2010
Palmitic acid	Leaves/roots	Chatterjee et al. 2010
Stearic acid	Roots	Misra et al. 2012
Vaccenic acid	Fruits	Mahrous et al. 2019
Vaccenoyl monoglyceride	Fruits	Mahrous et al. 2019
Coumarins		
Aesculetin	Fruit	Abou-Douh 2002

(Continued)

TABLE 1.1 (Continued)   Phytochemicals reported in *W. somnifera*

COMPOUND	PLANT PART	REFERENCE
Scopoletin	Fruit	Abou-Douh 2002; Sharma et al. 2013
Triterpenes		
β-Amyrin	Fruit	Abou-Douh 2002
Oleanolic acid	Roots	Misra et al. 2012
Phenyl propanoid esters		
Withaninsams A	Roots	Baek et al. 2019
Withaninsams B	Roots	Baek et al. 2019
Others		
Acetosyringone	Roots	Baek et al. 2019
Benzoic acid	Roots, leaves	Alam et al. 2011
Benzo[6:7]chroman	Roots	Anjaneyulu and Rao 1997
2,5-Dioxo-3-tetratriacont-3′-enyl-,4-dioxane	Roots	Misra et al. 2012
N-trans-Feruloyl methoxytyramine	Roots	Baek et al. 2019
N-trans-Feruloyltyramine	Roots	Baek et al. 2019
Octacosane	Roots	Misra et al. 2012
Squalene	Fruits	Bhatia et al. 2013
Tocopherol	Fruits	Bhatia et al. 2013

Ghosh 2015; Alam et al. 2016; Ahmad and Dar 2017; Kaul and Wadhwa 2017; Rayees and Malik 2017). Phytochemical composition, medicinal applications and nutrapharmaceutical potentials of WS have been reviewed recently (Saleem et al. 2020). WS is a potential source for the treatment of a wide range of diseases especially anxiety and other CNS disorders (Mukherjee et al. 2021).

It is also used to treat insomnia and Parkinson's and Alzheimer's diseases. It relieves stress, improves memory, sperm count and motility (Datta et al. 2011). It improves body's defence against chronic diseases by enhancing cell-mediated immunity, anti-inflammatory and antioxidant effects (Murthy et al. 2010). It works well for reducing anxiety and stress, enhancing performance, improving glucose metabolism and increasing testosterone levels. Several pre-clinical and clinical studies have been listed in a recent review on the use of WS for mental illnesses (Tandon and Yadav 2020). WS is considered an effective and safe ergogenic aid for improving the strength, endurance and recovery of athletes (Achini et al. 2020). WS is reported to act as a supplement for enhanced performance including increased muscle strength (Wankhede et al. 2015), boost in testosterone (Lopresti et al. 2019a) and improved VO_{2max} (Pérez-Gómez et al. 2020). WS supplementation was effective in improving variables related to strength/power, cardiorespiratory fitness and fatigue/recovery in healthy men and women (Bonilla et al. 2021). Supplementation with WS root extracts improved the maximum oxygen consumption (VO_{2max}) or the aerobic capacity of healthy adults and athletes (Pérez-Gómez et al. 2020).

There has been a notable increase in the pharmacological and clinical research of WS in the recent past and evidences for properties such as anti-inflammatory, antiarthritic, antiageing, antianxiety, antistress, neuroprotective, anticancer, adaptogenic and antidepressant are readily available in literature. There are several reviews on the pharmacological activities of WS (Mishra et al. 2000; Gupta and Rana 2007; Singh et al. 2010a, 2010b, 2011a; Vyas et al. 2011; Narinderpal et al. 2013; Tiwari et al. 2014; Bano et al. 2015; Dar et al. 2015, 2016; Halder and Ghosh 2015; Krutika et al. 2016; Ahmad and Dar 2017). The scope of immunomodulatory drugs in Ayurveda including WS for prevention and treatment of Covid-19 has been reviewed (Srivastava and Saxena 2020). It was recently reported that WS can bind to Covid-19 spike proteins thereby suggesting it to be a good therapeutic candidate for Covid-19 treatment (Kashyap et al. 2020). Withanone and withaferin A are predicted to block entry of SARS-CoV-2 into cells (Kumar et al. 2020). Withaferin A has also been suggested as a potential therapeutic agent against COVID-19 infection (Straughn and Kakar 2020).

1.4.2 Pharmacological Studies

A large number of studies have been carried out on the pharmacological and clinical activities of WS (Table 1.2). Antibacterial and antifungal activity of WS has been reviewed (Khanchandani et al. 2019). The water extract of the root powder orally fed to experimental rats was found to ameliorate the symptoms of induced arthritis (Khan et al. 2019). Significant antimycobacterial activity was observed with 70% methanol root extract (Adaikkappan et al. 2012). Animal studies confirmed the use of WS as an antistress adaptogen (Archana and Namasivayam 1999). Thyrotropic effect was confirmed in animal studies as WS methanolic extract treatment normalized thyroid indices (Abdel-Wahhab et al. 2019). In a recent review, the use of WS in diabetes has been discussed in detail (Durg et al. 2020). Treatment with WS reduced the elevated levels of blood glucose, HbA1c and insulin in the noninsulin-dependent diabetes mellitus (NIDDM) rats (Anwer et al. 2008). The blood-brain barrier permeability of withanamides in WS fruit extract was tested in mice using LC-QTOF-MS and results showed that the withanamides crossed the blood-brain barrier suggesting the use of WS fruit extract for stress-induced neurological disorders

TABLE 1.2 Pharmacological and clinical studies of *W. somnifera*

SR. NO.	DISEASE/ACTIVITY	REFERENCE PHARMACOLOGICAL STUDIES	CLINICAL STUDIES
1	Adaptogen	Bhattacharya and Muruganandam 2003	Salve et al. 2019
2	Adjuvant to chemotherapy		Biswal et al. 2013
3	Adrenal function		Powell et al. 2017
4	Alzheimer's disease	Jayaprakasam et al. 2010; Sehgal et al. 2012	
5	Analgesic activity	Dey et al. 2016	Murthy et al. 2019
6	Antiageing effect	Kumar et al. 2013; Raghuraman and Subramaniam 2016; Koval et al. 2021	
7	Antibacterial	Rohma et al. 2018; Khanchandani et al. 2019	
8	Anticholinesterase activity	Choudhary et al. 2004; Mahrous et al. 2019	
9	Antidepressant	Husain et al. 2007; Antony et al. 2020	Gannon et al. 2019
10	Antifungal	Khanchandani et al. 2019	
11	Anti-inflammatory	Rasool and Varalakshmi 2006; Gupta and Singh 2014	
12	Antileukemic	Sayantan and Sujata 2021	
13	Antilipidemic	Jayaprakasam et al. 2004	
14	Antimalarial	Dikasso et al. 2006	
15	Antimicrobial	Girish et al. 2006; Mwitari et al. 2013	
16	Antinociceptive and anti-inflammatory	Shahraki et al. 2016	
17	Antitussive	Sinha et al. 2011	
18	Antiviral	Jain et al. 2018	Keche et al. 2010
19	Antioxidant	Rohma et al. 2018	
20	Anxiety	Bhattacharya et al. 2000b; Kaur et al. 2017	Andrade et al. 2000; Pratte et al. 2014; Cooley et al. 2009
21	Arthritis	Khan et al. 2019	Kulkarni et al. 1991

(Continued)

TABLE 1.2 (Continued)   Pharmacological and clinical studies of *W. somnifera*

SR. NO.	DISEASE/ACTIVITY	REFERENCE PHARMACOLOGICAL STUDIES	REFERENCE CLINICAL STUDIES
22	Bone protection	Khedgikar et al. 2015	
23	Brain health	Tohda et al. 2005; Konar et al. 2011; Zahiruddin et al. 2020	
24	Cancer	Joshi 2017; Shah et al. 2018; Dutta et al. 2019	Biswal et al. 2013; Lee and Choi 2016
25	Chemotherapy-induced neutropenia in mice	Gupta et al. 2001	
26	Cognitive function in patients with bipolar disorder		Chengappa et al. 2013
27	Constipation		Singh and Rajoria 2018
28	Dementia	Kuboyama et al. 2006;	
29	Dermatological diseases	Farooqui et al. 2018; Bungau et al. 2021	
30	Diabetes	Anwer et al. 2008, 2012	Andallu and Radhika 2000
31	Endurance		Shenoy et al. 2012; Choudhary et al. 2015
32	Epilepsy	Raju et al. 2017	
33	Heart health	Mohanty et al. 2008	Sandhu et al. 2010
34	Hepatoprotective	Bhattacharya et al. 2000a; Mansour and Hafez 2012	
35	Huntington's disease	Kumar and Kumar 2009	
36	Hypocholesteromic effect	Visavadiya and Narasimhacharya 2007	
37	Hypolipidaemic	Udayakumar et al. 2009	
38	Hypothyroid	Abdel-Wahhab et al. 2019	Sharma et al. 2018
39	Immunomodulatory	Davis and Kuttan 2000	
40	Inflammatory bowel disease.	Pawar et al. 2011	
41	Ischemic stroke	Sood et al. 2016	

(Continued)

TABLE 1.2 (Continued)   Pharmacological and clinical studies of *W. somnifera*

SR. NO.	DISEASE/ACTIVITY	REFERENCE PHARMACOLOGICAL STUDIES	CLINICAL STUDIES
42	Kidney damage	Vedi et al. 2014	
43	Knee joint pain		Ramakanth et al. 2016
44	Leishmaniasis (Antiparasitic)	Grover et al. 2012; Kaur et al. 2014; Chandrasekaran et al. 2017	
45	Longevity	Akhoon et al. 2018	
46	Lung injury	Gao et al. 2015	
47	Lupus	Minhas et al. 2012	
48	Male fertility	Sengupta et al. 2018	Ahmad et al. 2011; Sengupta et al. 2018
49	Memory and cognitive function	Alzoubi et al. 2019	Chengappa et al. 2013; Choudhary et al. 2017a
50	Morphine dependence	Caputi et al. 2018; Bassareo et al. 2019	
51	Muscle strength and recovery		Wankhede et al. 2015
52	Nephroprotective	Govindappa et al. 2019	
53	Neuroinflammation	Gupta and Kaur 2019	
54	Neuroprotective	Shah et al. 2015; Birla et al. 2019	Pingali et al. 2014
55	Obsessive-compulsive disorder (OCD)	Kaurav et al. 2012	Jahanbakhsh et al. 2016
56	Osteoarthritis		Sumantran et al. 2007
57	Oxidative stress	Bhattacharya et al. 1997; Ahmed et al. 2013	Kuchewar et al. 2014
58	Parkinson's disease	Prakash et al. 2013; Singh et al. 2015b	
59	Rheumatoid arthritis		Kumar et al. 2015b
60	Schizophrenia		Chengappa et al. 2013; Marell and Brar 2017; Gannon et al. 2019

(Continued)

TABLE 1.2 (Continued) Pharmacological and clinical studies of *W. somnifera*

SR. NO.	DISEASE/ACTIVITY	REFERENCE PHARMACOLOGICAL STUDIES	CLINICAL STUDIES
61	Semen quality		Ahmad et al. 2010
62	Sexual function in men		Azgomi et al. 2018
63	Sexual function in Women		Dongre et al. 2015; Azgomi et al. 2018
64	Sleep	Kumar and Kalonia 2008; Kaushik et al. 2017	Langade et al. 2019; Deshpande et al. 2020; Kelgane et al. 2020
65	Snake venom	Machiah et al. 2006	
66	Stress	Archana and Namasivayam 1999; Bhattacharya and Muruganandam 2003; Gajarmal et al. 2014;	Choudhary et al. 2017b; Chandrasekhar et al. 2012; Lopresti et al. 2019b; Gannon et al. 2019
67	Testosterone level	Rahmati et al. 2016	Lopresti et al. 2019a
68	Tuberculosis	Adaikkappan et al. 2012	Debnath et al. 2012
69	Weight loss and muscle growth		Wankhede et al. 2015; Choudhary et al. 2017b

(Vareed et al. 2014). The neuroprotective properties of WS have been reviewed recently and preclinical as well as clinical studies suggest the use of WS against neurodegenerative diseases (Dar and Ahmad 2020; Zahiruddin et al. 2020). The WS is a potent neuroprotective agent playing a significant role in ameliorating the neurodegenerative disorder Parkinson's disease (Singh et al. 2010b). It protects against post-traumatic stress disorder (PTSD)-induced impairment of short- and long-term memory, possibly through antagonizing hippocampal oxidative stress (Alzoubi et al. 2019). It was found to provide neuroprotective activity against bisphenol A-induced oxidative stress and memory impairment in mice (Birla et al. 2019). A purified glycoprotein from WS has been found to inhibit halouronidase activity of snake venoms (Machiah et al. 2006). Treatment of sleep-deprived rats with water extract of WS leaves confirmed anxiolytic, anti-inflammatory and antiapoptopic properties (Kaur et al. 2017). Oral feeding of leaf water extract of WS prevented lipopolysaccharide-induced neuroinflammation, neurodegeneration, cognitive decline, impairments in synaptic plasticity and improved working memory and learning and locomotor coordination (Gupta and Kaur 2019).

Animal studies revealed that the antioxidant and antiapoptotic properties of WS contribute to the cardioprotective effects observed in WS-treated animals (Mohanty et al. 2008). A study of WS root extract on anxiety and depression in rats showed antidepressant effect supporting its use as mood enhancer (Husain et al. 2007). Chronic stress in rat model showed that WS has significant antistress adaptogenic activity (Bhattacharya and Muruganandam 2003). Withanolides in alcoholic fractions of WS demonstrated a potent antileishmanial and immunomodulatory activities in visceral leishmaniasis (Chandrasekaran et al. 2017). WS root powder acts as an anti-inflammatory and antioxidant agent decreasing arthritic effects in collagen-induced arthritic rats (Gupta and Singh 2014). The high anti-inflammatory activity of WS may be attributed to the biologically active steroids such as withaferin A (Khare 2007).

WS has been found to stimulate stem cell proliferation when used as an adjuvant during radiation therapy (Kuttan 1996). Several *in vitro* and animal studies have been conducted on the effect of WS on colon cancer, blood cancer, lung cancer, skin cancer, renal cancer, prostate cancer, pancreatic cancer, fibrosarcoma, melanoma, cervical cancer, osteosarcoma, breast cancer, brain cancer, head and neck and squamous cell sarcoma. WS root extract is a potent inhibitor of lipogenesis in prostate cancer cells (Kim et al. 2020). The anticancer activities of WS extract and its constituents have been reviewed recently (Winters 2006; Lee and Choi 2016; Palliyaguru et al. 2016; Rai et al. 2016; Joshi 2017; Shah et al. 2018; Dutta et al. 2019; Saggam et al. 2020; Sivasankarapillai et al. 2020). Various parts of WS, especially its roots, have been found to be effective against different kinds of cancers. Withanolides, withaferins, withanone and withanosides have been reported to be effective against different cancer cell lines (Rai et al. 2016). Anticarcinogenic effect in lung, breast, colon, cervical, brain, prostate and other cancers has been observed with the extracts of leaves, roots, stems and fruits as well as isolated withanolides (withaferin A) (Dutta et al. 2019). At least five signalling pathways are involved in the selective inhibition of cancer cells by WS (Joshi 2017). Withaferin A is an inhibitor of angiogenesis and thus protective against cancers (Mohan et al. 2004). Subcritical water extracts of WS and withaferin A showed significant reduction in cell viability of cervical cancer (HeLA) cell, with IC50 values of 10 mg/mL and 8.5 μM/mL, respectively (Nile et al. 2019). The antioxidant/ free radical scavenging activity of WS extract seems to be responsible for its potential to reduce tumour growth (Prakash et al. 2002). A recent review highlights the importance of WS in countering the potential oncogenic signalling mediators in a variety of cancer types (Mehta et al. 2020).

The active phytoconstituents are alkaloids, withanolides, withaferins, acylsteryl glucosides, glycowithanolides, flavonoids and phenolics. The curative properties of WS can be attributed mainly to withanolides and phenolics (Jamal et al. 1995; Budhiraja et al. 2000). Two main withanolides, withaferin A and withanolide D, contribute much of the pharmacological activity of WS (Mishra et al. 2000; Anonymous 2004). Acylsteryl glucosides (sitoindoside VII and VIII) in Ashwagandha are anti-inflammatory and antistress agents (Bhattacharya et al. 1987). Several withanolides showed promising pharamcological properties for the treatment of inflammation-mediated chronic diseases including arthritis, autoimmune, cancer and neurodegenerative diseases (White et al. 2016). A concise overview of the molecular mechanisms by which withaferin A orchestrates its anti-inflammatory effects to restore immune homeostasis is reported (Logie and Berghe 2020). Withaferin A and withanolide D possess significant antitumour and radiosensitizing properties (Singh et al. 2010b). Withasilolides A, B, D, F and withanone were found to be cytotoxic towards human cancer cell lines (Kim et al. 2019). Withanolide D decreased the suppression of apoptosis in mice and impaired the progression of the disease, so, we can conclude that withanolide D of Ashwagandha may hold a promise towards a new therapeutic strategy in leukemia (Sayantan and Sujata 2021). Withanamides are potent lipid peroxidation inhibitors (Jayaprakasam et al. 2004) and anti-Alzheimer's agent (Jayaprakasam et al. 2010). Proteins from WS such as glycoprotein and lectin like-protein possess potent therapeutic properties like antimicrobial, anti-snake venom poison and antimicrobial (Dar et al. 2016). A monomeric glycoprotein, *W. somnifera* glycoprotein, isolated from WS roots demonstrated antimicrobial activity (Girish et al. 2006). The withanolides in human body serve as hormone precursors able to convert into the required hormones as needed. It can also regulate physiological processes and serve as an adaptogen able to withstand stress, serve as an antioxidant and immunostimulator.

1.4.3 Clinical Studies

Several clinical studies have been reported on the therapeutic effects of WS (Pratte et al. 2014; Rayees and Malik 2017; Ng et al. 2020). The therapeutic adjuvant potential of WS in cancer management is highlighted (Saggam et al. 2020). A recent study demonstrated that an intake of the WS extract as a supplement for 8 weeks in healthy males aged between 40 and 70 years resulted in significant improvement in salivary dehydro epiandrosterone sulfate (DHEA-S) and testosterone thought to be associated with positive health-enhancing effects (Lopresti et al. 2019a). A double-blind study in children involving milk fortified with WS confirmed the growth-promoting effect of WS (Venkataraghavan et al. 1980). Another study on healthy males revealed general improvement of health along with improvement in their sexual performance (Bone 1996). Cognitive decline and memory loss are the accompanying problems of a greying popula-tion and clinical studies proved that WS supplementation improved cognition, agility and attention (Ng et al. 2020). For cardiovascular protection, WS exhib-ited hypoglycemic, diuretic and hypocholesteromic effects in human subjects. On treatment with WS root powder for 30 days, decrease in blood glucose level, increase in urine sodium, urine volume and decrease in serum cholesterol, tri-glycerides and low-density lipoproteins were observed (Andallu and Radhika 2000). Treatment of 60 infertile men for 3 months with WS root powder (5 g/day) resulted in a decrease in stress, improved the level of antioxidants and improved overall semen quality in a significant number of individuals (Ahmad et al. 2011). Another clinical study reports that WS root extract can be used for body weight management in adults under chronic stress (Choudhary et al. 2017b).

Enhancement of both immediate and general memory was observed in 50 adults with mild cognitive impairment (MCI) on treatment with WS root extract for 8 weeks (Choudhary et al. 2017a). Anxiety disorder treatment human trial with WS resulted in greater score improvements in anxiety or stress scales (Pratte et al. 2014). A randomized, double-blind, placebo-controlled study of WS extract in healthy adults demonstrated significant stress-relieving effects (Lopresti et al. 2019b). WS extract as an adjuvant to chemotherapy of breast cancer patients reduced fatigue and led to longer survival (Biswal et al. 2013). A herbal formula containing WS given to arthritic patients brought about reduction of the severity of pain and disability (Kulkarni et al. 1991). WS treatment on chronic stress sub-jects led to a reduction in all stress assessment scores on day 60 of the treatment (Chandrasekhar et al. 2012). Patients with ICD-10 anxiety disorders recorded significant reduction in anxiety level on treatment with ethanolic extract of WS (Andrade et al. 2000). A recent study revealed that *Withania* extract can improve cognitive and psychomotor performance (Pingali et al. 2014).

A clinical study of WS root extract in 50 patients with subclinical hypo-thyroidism demonstrated that WS root extract is beneficial in normalizing the thyroid indices (Sharma et al. 2018). An 8-week clinical study of high concentration WS root extract on 50 female subjects revealed that oral admin-istration of WS extract improves sexual function in healthy women (Dongre et al. 2015). Treatment with WS reduced oxidative stress and improved the level of antioxidants and improved semen quality in infertile men (Ahmad et al. 2010). WS was found to enhance spermatogenesis and sperm-related indices in male and sexual behaviours in female showing the effect of WS on reproductive system (Azgomi et al. 2018). Effect of WS on male fertil-ity has been reviewed (Teixeira and Duarte de Araujo 2019). Animal studies supported the use of WS as a mood stabilizer in clinical conditions of anxi-ety and depression (Bhattacharya et al. 2000b). A randomized, double-blind, placebo-controlled study involving 60 patients with insomnia treated with WS root extracts at a dose of 300 mg extract twice daily reported improved sleep quality and sleep onset latency without any side effects such as drug dependency (Langade et al. 2019).

1.5 PHYTOCHEMICAL ANALYSIS

W. somnifera (L.) Dunal (Solanaceae), known as Ashwagandha or Indian ginseng, is cultivated in India for centuries and used in more than 100 formulations (Gajbhiye et al. 2015). Natural products are routinely identified and analyzed by spectroscopic, chemical and chromatographic methods. Quantifying the phytochemical contents in herbs is an important step in assuring the quality and efficacy of herbal products. Many analytical techniques such as HPTLC, HPLC, NMR and LC-MS have been used for the qualitative and quantitative analysis of phytoconstituents in WS and its formulations for the last 50 years or more. Several convenient methods of quantification of WS components by HPTLC (Jirge et al. 2011; Patel et al. 2014; Tomar et al. 2019), HPLC (Ganzera et al. 2003; Ali et al. 2010), NMR (Chatterjee et al. 2010; Sidhu et al. 2011; Trivedi et al. 2017), GC-MS (Chatterjee et al. 2010; Sharma et al. 2013; Trivedi et al. 2017) and LC-MS (Khajuria et al. 2004; Musharraf et al. 2011; Bolleddula et al. 2012; Mirjalili et al. 2013; Gajbhiye et al. 2015; Filipiak-Szok et al. 2017; Trivedi et al. 2017) have been reported.

1.5.1 HPTLC

A validated HPTLC method is reported for the simultaneous determinations of three phenolic acids (caffeic acid, ferulic acid and benzoic acid) and three withanolides (withaferin A, withanone and withanolide A) from WS plants (root, stem and leaf) and its herbal products (Tomar et al. 2019). Simultaneous determination of withaferin A, 12-deoxywithastramonolide and withanolide A in WS plant samples by HPTLC is reported (Srivastava et al. 2008). Methanol extracts of the separated HPTLC bands of withaferin A, 12-deoxywithastramonolide and withanolide A (all having m. wt. 470) gave positive ion ESI mass spectra showing abundant $[M+Na]^+$ and $[M+H]^+$ ions at *m/z* 493 and 471, respectively (Srivastava et al. 2008).

1.5.2 HPLC

Several HPLC methods have been developed for the determination of a limited number of markers in WS (Bessalle and Lavie 1987; Bala et al. 2004). A routine HPLC-PDA method was developed and validated for the simultaneous identification and determination of withaferin A, 12-deoxy-withastramonolide, withanolide A, withanolide B, withanoside IV and withanoside V in WS raw materials and product samples (Penman et al. 2007). Simultaneous analysis of nine structurally similar withanolides was carried out using reversed-phase HPLC-PAD-ELSD method (Chaurasiya et al. 2008). Using the HPLC method developed for the simultaneous determination of flavonoid glycosides in aerial parts and roots of WS, three flavonoid glycosides were detected in aerial parts, but none in the roots (Mundkinajeddu et al. 2014). This is an important finding since it can be used to detect adulteration of root extract with extracts from aerial parts. Five phenolics and three flavonoids have been identified in the roots, fruits and leaves extracts of WS and catechin was found the highest in leaves by an HPLC method (Alam et al. 2011). HPLC analysis of methanol extracts of WS showed that higher quantities of withanolides were present in root compared to stem and rhizome head (Geetha et al. 2010). HPLC analysis of WS plants grown from seedling stage till 150 days showed that the contents of withanolide A and withaferin A were maximum at 60 days from germination (Nair and Praveen 2019). HPLC analysis of withaferin A and withanolide D in root, stem and leaf of WS showed that the stem contained the lowest percentage (0.055%) of withanolides (withaferin A and withanolide D), whereas the root and leaf contained 0.259% and 0.241%, respectively (Ganzera et al. 2003). Withaferin A and withanolide A in leaves and roots of WS have been analyzed by a validated RP-HPLC method (Sharma 2013). HPLC analysis revealed varied concentrations of withanolide A in different genotypes of WS (Chauhan et al. 2019). The genetic diversity of Iranian WS was studied using random amplified polymorphic DNA (RAPD) markers and their withaferin A content. Variations in the RAPD results and withaferin A content reflected the genetic factors and geographic distribution and withaferin A was found higher in the aerial part than in the root by HPLC (Mirjalili et al. 2009b). Wide variations in the contents of the seven tested constituents were observed in several mono- and polyherbal formulations available in India, thus emphasizing the need for standardization and quality control (Sangwan et al. 2004). From a study of the chemical variation in 25 collections of Indian WS, it was concluded that phytochemical variations are by and large gene-related (Kumar et al. 2007). HPLC analysis of wild and cultivated plant types of WS showed that withaferin A, withanolide A and 12-deoxywithastramonolide were present in both the wild and the cultivated types with quantitative differences and the tested constituents were several times greater in some plants of the wild type (Joshi et al. 2010). HPLC analysis of withaferin A, withanolide A and 12-deoxywithastramonolide in 53 genotypes of WS collected from different geographical regions of India showed significant differences in the contents between the accessions (Srivastava et al. 2018). Simultaneous quantification of nine structurally similar withanolides (withanolides A, B, IV, V, withanone, 27- hydroxywithanone, withaferin A, withastramonolide and physagulin D) from the roots of Egyptian WS using HPLC was reported (Ismail 2013). A simple and rapid HPLC method was developed for the quantification of withaferin A, 12-deoxywithastromonolide and withanolide A in WS plant extracts and formulations (Kumar et al. 2018). Five varieties of Ashwagandha (*W. somnifera*) i.e. Chetak, Pratap, Nimitli, Poshita and Jawahar 20 were analyzed for withanolide A and withaferin A in leaf, stem, root and seeds using HPLC. Their contents varied from tissue to tissue and variety to variety (Singh et al. 2018a).

1.5.3 NMR

Seventeen metabolites were identified and quantified in nonpolar and polar extracts of different fruit development stages of WS by NMR spectroscopy (Sidhu et al. 2011). These investigations also revealed the metabolic alterations in the fruits of WS at different stages of development and that the content of withanolides decreases in mature fruits while that of withanamide increases. The results indicated specific stages when fruits can be harvested for obtaining bioactive compounds of desired pharmacological activity (Sidhu et al. 2011). Metabolic characterization of WS leaves, stems and roots collected from six different regions in India using ¹H NMR was reported (Namdeo et al. 2011). This study revealed the presence of two groups of withanolides: 4-OH and 5,6-epoxy withanolides (withaferin A-like steroids) and 5-OH and 6,7-epoxy withanolides (withanolide A-like steroids). Their ratio in leaf could discriminate the samples from different regions. Using HR-MAS NMR, 41 metabolites were detected from root and leaf tissues of WS (Bharti et al. 2011). The important metabolites withaferin A and withanone showed distinctive quantitative variability among the four chemotypes. GC-MS and ¹H NMR analysis revealed 82 metabolites including acids, aromatic amino acids, sugars, sugar alcohols, polyols, tocopherols, sterols and withanamides in WS fruits (Bhatia et al. 2013). Their variations were studied in fruits from four different chemotypes of WS. Metabolic profiling of WS using HPLC, NMR and GC-MS led to the identification of 62 primary and secondary metabolites from WS leaves and 48 from roots (Chatterjee et al. 2010). NMR analysis revealed that withaferin A and withanone were the major metabolites in the chloroform fraction of leaves, whereas withanolide A and withanone were the major metabolites in the roots. Butanolic fraction of the leaf indicated the presence of physagulin, withanoside IV and withanoside VI. Butanol fraction of roots indicated the presence of withanoside IV and withanoside VI (Chatterjee et al. 2010).

1.5.4 Applications of Mass Spectrometry in *Withania Somnifera* Research

There is enhanced scope of metabolic identification and quantification now due to the recent advancements and refinements in analytical mass spectrometry. Applications of these advancements in the metabolomics of WS are reviewed (Tetali et al. 2021). GC-MS and LC-MS techniques are more often used for the structural identification of phytoconstituents from WS. GC-MS is employed for nonpolar or derivatized polar molecules, whereas LC-MS is generally more suitable for medium polar to polar molecules.

1.5.4.1 GC-MS

A comprehensive GC-MS analysis of the leaf and root extracts of WS was reported (Chatterjee et al. 2010). Four fractions of different polarities (*n*-hexane, aqueous methanol, chloroform and *n*-butanol) were prepared from the leaf and root samples of WS and subjected to GC-MS analysis. GC-MS of the *n*-hexane extract after esterification (methyl ester) revealed that palmitic acid and linolenic acid were the predominant fatty acids in the leaves, whereas palmitic acid and linoeic acid were the predominant fatty acids in the roots. The $CHCl_3$ and *n*-butanol fractions were analyzed by GC-MS after preparation of the trimethyl silyl (TMS) derivatives. 1-Octanol, different aromatic alcohols, aromatic acids and β-sitosterol were among the 14 components detected. The TMS derivatives of the aqueous fraction on GC-MS indicated the presence of fructose, galactose, N-acetyl glucosamine, myo-inositol, glycerol, GABA and malic acid (Chatterjee et al. 2010). A GC-MS method was developed to analyze the alkaloid content of methanolic extracts of roots and callus of WS and the results revealed that 17 alkaloids were present and withasomnine was the main alkaloid in roots and callus, but the content of tropane alkaloids is higher in roots than callus (Sharma et al. 2013). Metabolic profiling of the hydroalcoholic extract of WS roots using GC-MS, LC-MS and NMR spectroscopy led to the identification of 43 withanolides including the first-time identified dihydrowithanolide D and ixocarpalactone A (Trivedi et al. 2017).

GC-MS of the volatile oil of leaves and stems of WS growing in Albaha region Saudi Arabia indicated the presence of 36 compounds including alcohols, hydrocarbons, aromatics, aldehydes and ketones (Ali et al. 2020). The acetone insoluble fraction of the methanol extract of leaves and stems showed the presence of three *n*-hydrocarbons with *n*-pentacosane (n-$C_{25}H_{52}$) as the major component in leaves while in stems there are six compounds in which nonacosane(n-$C_{29}H_{60}$) was the major component. The unsaponifiable matter in the leaves and stems contained hydrocarbons, alcohols, aldehydes and ketones. Two steroids ergost-5-en-3-ol and stigmasterol and a triterpene α-amyrin were present in the unsaponifiable matter from the seeds. GC-MS data of the methyl esters of fatty acids from WS leaves, stem and seeds showed the presence of 17 fatty acids in varying amounts (Ali et al. 2020). Using GC-MS 29 metabolites was identified in methanol extracts of *in vitro* cultured and field grown roots of WS (Senthil et al. 2015).

1.5.4.2 LC-MS

Structural elucidation and gas-phase fragmentation of ten withanolides were studied using positive ion ESI-QTOF-MS/MS. The [M+H]$^+$ ions fragmented by multiple losses of H_2O and C-17 substituted lactone moiety. Structure-fragmentation relationships were proposed in an attempt to identify withanolides in WS plant extracts using LC-MS (Musharraf et al. 2011). Withanolides possessing hydroxyl groups at C-4, C-5, C-17, C-20 and C-27 and an epoxy group at C-5/C-6 and C-6/C-7 were evaluated by ESI-QqTOF-MS/MS. A general strategy was developed for the rapid identification of withanolides based on their MS/MS fragmentation (Figure 1.1). Loss of the side chain containing

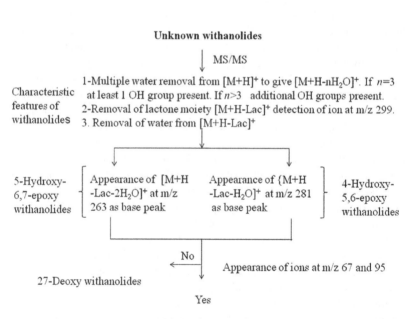

FIGURE 1.1   General strategy for the rapid identification of withanolides by ESI-QqTOF-MS/MS (with permission from Musharraf et al. 2011).

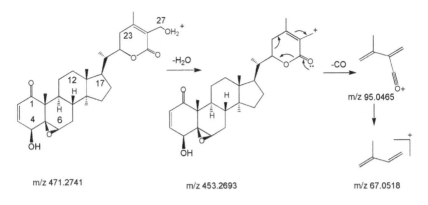

FIGURE 1.2 Proposed scheme CID-MS/MS fragmentation pathway of the precursor ion at *m/z* 471.2741 that yields the product ions at *m/z* 67 and 95 (with permission from Musharraf et al. 2011).

the lactone ring followed by loss of one or two molecules of water is the preferred fragmentation retaining the charge on the ergostane fragment. Charge retention in the lactone part leads to the cleavage of the lactone ring resulting to the ions at *m/z* 95 and *m/z* 67 (Figure 1.2). Similar fragmentations were also reported for withaferin A, 12-deoxywithastramonolide and withanolide (Gajbhiye et al. 2015).

Based on LC-MS and GC-MS investigations of the ethanol and methanol extracts of WS statistically significant (by Q score, retention peak threshold and PCA) substances were indicated according to literature and databases (Witter et al. 2020). An effective LC-HRMS method has been developed for online profiling and characterization of bioactive constituents present in the fruits of WS with an Orbitrap high resolution mass spectrometer. Glycosides yielded diagnostic fragment ions due to loss of the glycoside unit leading to the characterization of the aglycone unit. The 62 metabolites identified included 32 withanamides, 22 withanolides, 3 steroidal saponins, 2 lignanamides, feruloyl tyramine, methoxy feruloyl tyramine and a diglucoside of hydroxy palmitic acid (Bolleddula et al. 2012).

Withaferin A, 12-deoxywithastramonolide, withanolide A and withanone were estimated in WS plant extract samples using LC-MS in selected ion mode (SIM) detecting [M+Na]+ ions in the concentration range of 1.50 μg/mL to 6.5 μg/mL (Khajuria et al. 2004). The main withanolide withaferin A in WS extract was quantified by HPLC-MS/MS method (Mirjalili et al. 2013). The accumulation of withaferin A, 12-deoxywithastramonolide and withanolide A in root, stem, fruit and leaf of WS was monitored by quantifying their contents using a triple quadrupole LC-ESI-MS/MS (Gajbhiye et al. 2015). These three molecules had the same molecular weights, but their separation was achieved by LC and quantified by unique multiple reaction monitoring (MRM) transitions (m/z 471.2→281.1; m/z 471.2→175.1) for withaferin A (LOD: 3.33 ng/mL), (m/z 471.3→263.1; m/z 471.3→265.1) for 12-deoxywithastramonolide (LOD: 3.33 ng/mL) and (m/z 471.3→263.2; m/z 471.1→289.0) for withanolide A (LOD: 6.67 ng/mL). The content of withaferin A was the highest in leaves, whereas the contents of 12-deoxywithastramonolide and withanolide A were the highest in root (Gajbhiye et al. 2015). Simultaneous determination of phenolic acids, flavonols and alkaloids in alcoholic extract of powdered plant materials and standard dietary supplements of WS were carried out using LC-MS/MS and aflatoxins were determined by HPLC (Filipiak-Szok et al. 2017). The alkaloids were detected in positive ion ESI and flavonols and phenolic acids were detected in negative ion ESI mode. Seven flavonols, six phenolic acids and nine alkaloids (three each of purine, indole and isoquinoline) were identified in WS samples (Filipiak-Szok et al. 2017). LC-MS analysis of the methanol extract of WS roots resulted in the identification of six new withanolides, namely withasilolides A–F (Kim et al. 2019). Withaferin A was quantified in rat plasma and tissue following intravenous administration by LC-MS/MS in MRM mode using the transitions m/z 471.1 → 281 for withaferin A and m/z 488.1 → 263 for the internal standard withanolide A (Wang et al. 2019). Using a triple quadrupole MS/MS quantification of withaferin A in WS plant extracts was also reported by Mirjalili et al. (2013). MRM transitions m/z 471.2→281.1 and m/z 471.2→175.1 were used for quantification and confirmation, respectively. The achieved limit of detection (LOD) in the standards was 0.6 ng/mL and in plant extracts it was 6 ng/g. A selective HPLC-ESI-MS/MS method was developed for the simultaneous determination of withaferin A and withanolide A in mice plasma using the MRM transitions m/z 471.3 → 281.2 for withaferin A and m/z 488.3 → 263.1 for withanolide A with LOQs of 0.484 ng/mL and 0.476 ng/mL for withaferin A and withanolide A, respectively (Patil et al. 2013). Simultaneous quantification of 11 compounds (withanoside IV, withanoside VII, withanoside V, withaferin A, 12-deoxywithastramonolide, withanolide A, withanone, withanolide B, viscosalactone B, 27-hydroxywithanone and dihydrowithaferin A) in the alcoholic extract of WS roots by a novel UHPLC-PDA method was recently reported (Girme et al. 2020). The withanolides and withanosides were confirmed by UHPLC-ESI-MS/MS, some in the positive ion mode and the rest in negative ion mode.

1.5.4.3 MALDI TOF MS

Application of MALDI TOF mass spectrometry in natural products analysis was reviewed (Silva et al. 2016). Probing of metabolites in finely powdered plant samples by direct laser desorption mass spectrometry was attempted for WS. Withaferin A was characterized in WS leaves by laser desorption mass spectrometry followed by MS/MS (Musharraf et al. 2014). Protein profiles were analyzed by two-dimensional electrophoresis and MALDI TOF MS (Nagappan et al. 2012). MALDI TOF MS analysis of 2-DE protein spots from *in vitro* and *in vivo* grown root samples of WS revealed a high level of similarity in protein spots in both *in vitro* and *in vivo* root samples (Senthil et al. 2011). An effective strategy to combat the WS leaf pathogen *Alternaria alternata*, which is responsible for the biodeterioration of pharmaceutically important metabolites in WS, was developed using MALDI TOF MS. The differentially expressed proteins (38) were identified by MALDI TOF/TOF MS/MS to evaluate the modifications that take place at the proteomic level during compatible host pathogen interactions (Singh et al. 2017). Proteome analyses of tissues (seeds and leaves) of WS yielded 82 protein spots from seeds and 85 from leaves. Peptide mass fingerprinting using MALDI TOF MS led to the identification of 70 individual proteins from seeds and 74 from leaves. A comparative analysis showed that some proteins involved in housekeeping were common to both tissues, whereas some were exclusively tissue-specific (Dhar et al. 2012).

1.6 ADULTERATION

In India the estimated production of WS is 8429 metric tons, whereas the annual requirement is 9127 metric tons (Shrivastava and Sahu 2013). Both wild and cultivated WS with varying phytochemical contents are available in the market. The roots, stem, leaves and fruits have medicinal applications, but again the phytochemical contents vary widely. It is therefore very essential to have a standardized supply of herbal materials to ascertain the efficacy and quality of WS plant materials and finished products. Traditionally, the part used is the dried roots in powder form and currently they are also supplied in the form of an extract to herbal products and supplement manufacturers. As mentioned in traditional Ayurvedic medicine most manufacturers make their own extracts from the roots. Some proprietary WS formulations are appropriately labelled to contain the extracts of aerial parts, leaves or combinations of roots and other plant parts. It is adulteration to include undisclosed nonroot parts of WS, such as leaves, stem and aerial parts, which are rich in withaferin A and other withanolides. Aerial parts can be collected easily and more frequently than roots and that is motivation enough for adulteration. For determining the quality of herbal materials and their finished products, several chemical and phytochemical tests, analytical techniques and hyphenated analytical tests are used (Balekundri and Mannur 2020). Adulteration can be detected by techniques such as microscopic (Atal et al. 1975), macroscopic (Shalini et al. 2017), HPTLC and HPLC (Mundkinajeddu et al. 2014). The presence of three flavonoid glycosides quercetin 3-O-robinobioside-7-O-glucoside, quercetin 3-O-rutinoside-7-O-glucoside and kaempferol 3-O-robinobioside-7-O-glucoside which occur only in the aerial parts of WS is also a confirmation that WS root is adulterated with aerial parts. These flavonoid glycosides should be <0.01% for powdered root, and <0.04% for extracts (Singh et al. 2010b). It is of prime importance to ensure the quality of herbs and herbal products.

1.7 TOXICITY

Like most herbal supplements WS is considered safe for consumption without much side effects. Several cases of liver toxicity resulting from commercially available WS products have been reported recently (Philips et al. 2020). A case series presents a total of five cases of liver injury (two from Iceland and three from the United States) attributed to the intake of WS-containing supplements, with symptoms such as jaundice, nausea, lethargy, abdominal discomfort and prolonged pruritus and hyperbilirubinemia (Björnsson et al. 2020). When discontinued the toxicity symptoms resolve. It was later reported that withanone, a major metabolite of WS, forms adducts in DNA and interferes with its biological property, thus providing a potential mechanism for the reported liver damage (Siddiqui et al. 2021).

Quantitative Determination of Six Withanolides in Five Varieties of *W. Somnifera* Grown under Different Soil Treatment Conditions

---

2.1 INTRODUCTION

It was reported long back that WS showed chemogenetic variation showing morphological similarity, but differing in the contents of the chemical constituents (Abraham et al. 1968). *W. somnifera* (WS) has been divided into various chemotypes (accessions) based on the difference in withanolides. Analysis of 15 accessions of WS revealed that withanolides differed widely both qualitatively and quantitatively (Dhar et al. 2006). The nature of withanolides and their contents are known to be different in various chemotypes (Kalra and Kaushik 2017). It was also shown that the accessions of the Indian population of WS clustered

DOI: 10.1201/9781003186274-2

together with respect to their withanolide profile resulting in withaferin A-, with-anone-, withanolide D- or withanolide A-rich groups (Chaurasiya et al. 2009). A recent study describes the genetic variability, associations and path analysis of chemical and morphological traits in WS (Srivastava et al. 2018).

Farmers face several constraints such as limited land and water resources and small land holdings to allow medicinal plant cultivation in normal agricultural land. Allowing cultivation of medicinal plants in degraded and salt-affected lands is a viable proposition. Medicinal plants have the ability to tolerate ambient levels of salinity in soil (Dagar and Tomar 2006). The quality and content of principal phytocomponents are not affected by salinity or alkalinity (Kalaichelvi and Swaminathan 2009). In order to understand the effect of soil conditions on the phytoconstituents of WS we decided to analyze multi markers in leaf, stem and root of five varieties of WS grown under different soil conditions. Various analytical methods, including high performance thin layer chromatography (HPTLC) (Sharma et al. 2007; Patel et al. 2014), high performance liquid chromatography (HPLC) (Ganzera et al. 2003; Chaurasiya et al. 2008; Ali et al. 2010) and liquid chromatography-mass spectrometry (LC-MS) (Khajuria et al. 2004; Bolleddula et al. 2012; Mirjalili et al. 2013; Patil et al. 2013 Gajbhiye et al. 2015), have been reported for the quantification of a few of the major phytoconstituents of WS. We have developed and validated an efficient, rapid and sensitive ultra performance liquid chromatography-electrospray ionization-mass spectrometry/mass spectrometry (UPLC-ESI-MS/MS) method in the multiple reaction monitoring (MRM) acquisition mode for the simultaneous determination of six withanolides from the root, stem and leaf of WS. Using this method six marker compounds, namely withaferin A, withanolide A, withanolide B, withanone, withanoside IV and withanoside V in five varieties WS (root, stem and leaf) grown under six different soil conditions were quantified simultaneously (Chandra et al. 2016). Further, the developed method was applied for the simultaneous quantification of these markers in 26 different polyherbal marketed formulations of WS. Chemometric methods such as Hierarchical Cluster Analysis (HCA) and Principal Component Analysis (PCA) were employed to classify and evaluate the different samples.

2.2 MATERIALS AND METHODS

2.2.1 Reagents and Reference Standards

Methanol (LC–MS grade), acetonitrile (LC–MS grade) and formic acid (analytical grade) were purchased from Fluka, Sigma-Aldrich (St. Louis, MO, USA).

Milli-Q Ultra-pure water was obtained from a Millipore water purification system (Millipore, Milford, MA, USA). The reference standards (purity ≥90%) witha-ferin A, withanolide A, withanolide B, withanone, withanoside IV and withano-side V were purchased from Natural Remedies Pvt. Ltd., Bangalore, India.

2.2.2 Plant Material and Sample Collection

Five varieties of WS, namely NMITLI-101, NMITLI-108,NMITLI-118, NMITLI-135 and Poshita, were cultivated at different pH at Banthra Research Station of NBRI, Lucknow, India. Root, stem and leaf of the plant were dried at room temperature and ground to a fine powder. For sodicity evaluation of WS, soil was artificially created for different sodicity levels using sodium bicarbonate (NaHCO$_3$). The physicochemical properties of the experimental soil and dif-ferent soil treatment conditions and the finally recorded pH, electrical conduc-tivity (EC) and exchangeable sodium percent (ESP) of the artificially created soils are shown in Table 2.1. Twenty-six different polyherbal marketed formula-tions of WS manufactured by different pharmaceutical companies in different dosage forms, i.e., tablets and capsules, were purchased from local drug stores, Lucknow, UP, India as summarized in Table 2.2 (Chandra et al. 2016).

2.2.3 Extraction and Sample Preparation

2.2.3.1 Plant material

Soxhlet extraction was carried out in ethanol using 10 g of the sample pow-der (root, stem and leaf separately) for 6 h till the extract became colorless. Using a rotavapour at 55°C under reduced pressure at 20–50 kPa, the solvent was evaporated off and the residue kept in a desiccator. The dried extract (1 mg) was accurately weighed and dissolved in 1 mL of 100% methanol using ultrasonicator (Bandelin SONOREX, Berlin), filtered through 0.22 μm syringe filter (Millex-GV, PVDF, Merck Millipore, Darmstadt, Germany) and the filtrate diluted with methanol to a final working concentration in the range of 100 to 1000 ppb and 5 μL aliquot was injected into the UPLC–MS/MS system for analysis.

2.2.3.2 Polyherbal formulation

After completely removing the coating of herbal formulation (tablet form), a subsample (approximately 0.5 g) of each herbal formulation was placed in methanol (50 mL) at 26°C–28°C and sonicated for 30 min. After centrifugation

TABLE 2.1 Physicochemical properties of the experimental soil and different soil treatment condition for *W. somnifera*

PHYSICOCHEMICAL PROPERTIES OF THE SOIL		DIFFERENT SOIL TREATMENT CONDITION FOR W. SOMNIFERA			
		TREATMENT	*pH*	*EC dSm^{-1}*	*ESP*
Organic carbon (g kg^{-1})	3.9	T_1	8.2	0.4	10
Bulk density (Mg m³)	1.36	T_2	8.5	0.5	13
Particle density (Mg m³)	2.63	T_3	8.8	0.6	17
Porosity (%)	48.29	T_4	9.0	0.7	25
Sand (%)	25.15	T_5	9.3	0.8	30
Silt (%)	58.75	T_6	9.6	0.8	35
Clay (%)	16.1				
Soil texture	Silt loam				
Water holding capacity (%)	36.84				
CEC (c mol kg^{-1})	21.74				
Available N (kg ha^{-1})	95.3				
Available P (kg ha^{-1})	23.5				
Available K (kg ha^{-1})	280				
DTPA extractable Zn (mg kg^{-1})	0.62				
DTPA extractable Fe (mg kg^{-1})	36.4				
DTPA extractable Mn (mg kg^{-1})	6.84				
DTPA extractable Cu (mg kg^{-1})	1.24				

Source: With permission from Chandra et al. 2016.
CEC: Cation-exchange capacity, DTPA: diethylenetriaminepentaacetic acid, EC: electrical conductivity, ESP: exchangeable sodium percent

at 15,000 rpm for 10 min, the supernatant was filtered through a 0.22-μm syringe filter (Millex-GV, PVDF, Merck Millipore, Darmstadt, Germany). The filtrates were diluted with methanol to prepare working concentrations for the analysis.

2.2.3.3 Preparation of standard solutions

Approximately 1 mg of the six standards (withaferin A, withanolide A, withanolide B, withanone, withanoside IV and withanoside V) were accurately weighed and dissolved in 1 mL methanol separately. Exactly 100 μL of each

TABLE 2.2   Details of 26 marketed formulations

SAMPLE CODE	BRAND NAME	BATCH	MFG. DATE (MONTH/YEAR)	DOSAGE FORM
F-1	Collasyn	PAT 01	May-13	Tablet
F-2	Brento Forte	FH 004	Sep-14	Tablet
F-3	Nutritone	NTN 121401	Dec-14	Tablet
F-4	Vantak	0080	Jun-13	Tablet
F-5	Count Plus	0I1Q	Sep-14	Tablet
F-6	Myostaal Forte	SF071309	Aug-13	Tablet
F-7	Ulceromed	PS	Feb-13	Tablet
F-8	Femicron	FN-392	Nov-14	Capsule
F-9	Reserpento	C-1143	Jun-14	Tablet
F-10	Imunocin	AB15001	Jan-15	Tablet
F-11	Vigoroyal-F	VFMT002	Sep-13	Tablet
F-12	Flex-Imac Forte	FFC 025	Feb-14	Capsule
F-13	Vigoroyal-M	VMMT002	Nov-13	Tablet
F-14	Vantak-T	0102	Apr-14	Tablet
F-15	Calciplus	FM 22	Jan-15	Tablet
F-16	Prosticon	0036	Mar-14	Capsule
F-17	Kardotop	B-301	Aug-14	Tablet
F-18	Stresscom	BDO381	Dec-14	Tablet
F-19	Ashwagandha	72500321	May-15	Capsule
F-20	Confido	37400430B	Mar-14	Tablet
F-21	Gariforte	37500375	Feb-15	Tablet
F-22	Reosto	37500022	Jan-15	Tablet
F-23	Tentex Forte	37400826B	May-14	Tablet
F-24	Oxitard	37401337	Aug-14	Capsule
F-25	Abana	37400156B	Jan-14	Tablet
F-26	Speman	37400750B	May-14	Tablet

Source: With permission from Chandra et al. 2016.

individual standard solution was mixed and made up with methanol to 1 mL so the concentration of mixture was 100 ppm or 100 µg/mL for each standard. This 100 ppm stock solution was further diluted in range of 0.5 to 1000 ppb or 0.5 to 1000 ng/mL. So the working standard solutions were prepared by diluting the mixed standard solution with methanol to a series of concentrations that is used for plotting the calibration curves within the ranges from 0.5 to 1000 ng/mL. All stock and individual standard solutions were stored at −20°C until use and sonicated prior to injection.

2.2.4 Instrumentation

2.2.4.1 UPLC-QTRAP MS

The UPLC–MS analysis was carried out on a Waters ACQUITY UPLC™ system (Waters, Milford, MA, USA) interfaced with hybrid linear ion trap triple-quadrupole mass spectrometer (API 4000QTRAP™MS/MS system from AB Sciex, Concord, ON, Canada) equipped with electrospray (Turbo V) ion source. The Waters ACQUITY UPLC™ system was equipped with a binary solvent manager, sample manager, column oven and PDA. All the statistical calculations related to quantitative analysis were performed on Graph Pad Prism software version 5.

2.2.4.2 UPLC conditions

Chromatographic separation was performed on a Waters ACQUITY BEH™ C18 column (2.1 mm × 50 mm, 1.7 μm) operated at 25°C using gradient mobile phase consisting of 0.1% formic acid in water (A) and acetonitrile (B) at a flow rate of 0.3 mL/min. The gradient programme started with an initial linear increase from 30% to 90% B over 0 to 1.8 min, followed by a hold of 90% B from 1.8 min to 2.5 min and then back to the initial condition of 30% B from 2.5 min to 4.5 min. The sample injection volume was 5 μL.

2.2.4.3 MS conditions

Full scan mass spectra were recorded in the range *m/z* 100–1000. Nitrogen was used as the nebulizer, heater, and curtain gas as well as the collision-activated dissociation (CAD) gas. The optimized parameters for positive mode were as follows: the ion spray voltage was set to 5500 V; the turbospray temperature, 500°C; nebulizer gas (gas 1), 50 psi; heater gas (gas 2), 50 psi; collision gas, medium; the curtain gas (CUR), 20 psi. Nitrogen was used as the CAD gas and set as medium, and the interface heater was on. Quantitative analysis was performed using MRM acquisition mode and its conditions were optimized for each compound during infusion. Analyst 1.5.1 software package (AB Sciex) was used for instrument control and data acquisition. The MRM transitions and optimized compound-dependent MRM parameters: declustering potential (DP), entrance potential (EP), collision energy (CE), cell exit potential (CXP) for each analyte are listed in Table 2.3.

TABLE 2.3 Compound-dependent MRM parameters and transitions for each reference analyte (with permission from Chandra et al. 2016)

COMPOUND	RT (MIN)	Q1 MASS (Da)	Q3 MASS (Da)	DP	EP	CE	CXP
					MRM PARAMETERS		
Withanoside-IV	0.81	800.5	459.5	59	7	30	25
Withanoside-V	1.18	784.5	443.5	66	7	30	7
Withaferin-A	1.23	471	281.0	104	7	26	8
Withanone	1.44	488.3	263.2	63	6	26	13
Withanolide-A	1.45	488.3	262.9	81	7	28	13
Withanolide-B	1.85	472.4	455.2	83	5	19	24

Source: With permission from Chandra et al. 2016.
RT: retention time, DP: declustering potential, EP: entrance potential, CE: collision energy, CXP: cell exit potential

2.2.5 Multivariate Analysis

All the multivariate experiments were done using the software STATISTICA 7.0. The values were considered zero when the contents of the investigated compounds were below the quantitation limit or not detected in the samples (Chandra et al. 2015). HCA and PCA are the two unsupervised algorithms used to reveal unseen structures in the data. These methods permit distinction of relationships among different data points (i.e. samples) as well as among dissimilar variables. In this experiment, HCA of 26 formulations from different companies was performed, in which a method called average linkage between groups was employed and six markers were selected for the measurement. Similarly, PCA was carried out based on the contents of bioactive compounds.

2.3 METHOD DEVELOPMENT

2.3.1 Optimization of Chromatography and MS/MS Conditions

The chromatographic conditions, such as mobile phase composition, gradient elution procedure, column, flow rate and column temperature were optimized to achieve good separation within a short analysis time. Different types of columns, including ACQUITY BEH™ C18 column (2.1 mm × 50 mm, 1.7 μm) and ACQUITY CSH™ C18 (2.1 mm ×100 mm, 1.7 μm), were tested and compared. The results showed that although the ACQUITY CSH column could separate all compounds satisfactorily, ACQUITY BEH™ C18 column produced chromatograms with better peak shape and resolution in a shorter analysis time. Hence, Waters ACQUITY BEH™ C18 column (2.1 mm × 50 mm, 1.7 μm) was selected. On the basis of several trials using different mobile phases, including methanol–water, acetonitrile–water, acetonitrile–0.1% formic acid in water and methanol–0.1% formic acid in water the combination acetonitrile–0.1% formic in water was selected as the most appropriate mobile phase for the separation of the six compounds in 2.5 min runtime at a flow rate of 0.3 mL min⁻¹ and column temperature of 25°C.

The reference standards were infused separately by flow injection analysis (FIA) into the mass spectrometer, the precursor ion and product ions were acquired in positive ion modes. The six reference components (withanolide A, withanolide B, withaferin A, withanone, withanoside IV and withanoside V) exhibited the expected quasimolecular ion $[M+H]^+$ and adduct ion $[M+NH_4]^+$ (Khajuria et al. 2004). MRM parameters DP, EP, CE and CXP were optimized to achieve the most abundant, specific and stable MRM transition for each marker compound as shown in Table 2.3 and the MS/MS spectra shown in Figure 2.1. MRM-extracted ion chromatograms of the reference analytes are shown in Figure 2.2 (Chandra et al. 2016).

2.3.2 Validation

The developed UPLC-MRM method for quantitative analysis was validated according to the guidelines of the International Conference on Harmonization (ICH, Q2R1) by determining linearity, lower limit of detection (LOD), lower limit of quantification (LOQ), precision, solution stability and recovery.

2.3.2.1 Linearity, sensitivity and accuracy

LOD and LOQ under the present chromatographic conditions were determined by the calibration curve method: LOD = 3.3 × Sy.x/S; LOQ = 10 × Sy.x/S, where Sy.x = the standard deviation of residuals from line and S = the slope of the calibration curve. Calibration curves were prepared by plotting the peak area of marker compounds against the corresponding concentrations. The regression lines were linear in the concentration range studied and

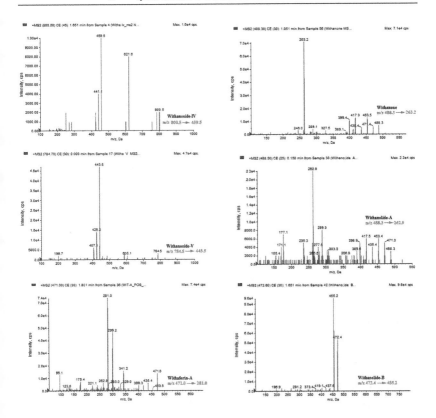

FIGURE 2.1 MS/MS spectra of selected six reference analytes (with permission from Chandra et al. 2016).

the corresponding coefficients of correlation are shown in Table 2.4. A good linear relationship with r^2 in the range of 0.9989–0.9998 was demonstrated for each analyte. The values of LOD and LOQ were investigated by analysis of working standard solutions prepared by dilution to a series of concentrations at detection limit, quantitation limit and in the nearby range as suggested from calibration curve extrapolation. The results of LOD and LOQ were confirmed by signal-to-noise ratio (S/N) of 3:1 and 10:1, respectively. The LOD for the six compounds ranged from 0.10 to 2.5 ng/mL and LOQ ranged from 0.30 to 8.0 ng/mL, as shown in Table 2.4. The accuracy of the analytical method was evaluated using the recovery test. The recovery tests of this method were studied by spiking a known quantity of the reference samples. Three different concentration levels (high, middle and low) of the analytical standards were added into the samples in triplicate and average

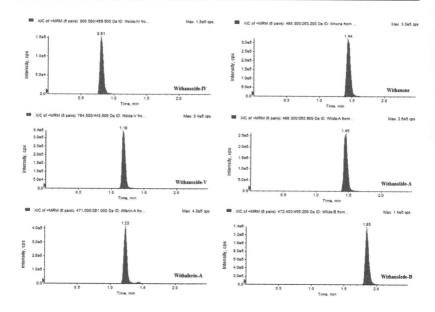

FIGURE 2.2   UPLC-MRM extracted ion chromatogram of selected six reference analytes (with permission from Chandra et al. 2016).

recoveries were determined. The mean recoveries ranged from 97.8% to 101.9% with relative standard deviation (RSD) less than 2.45% for the six reference compounds.

2.3.2.2 *Precision and stability*

The precision of the developed method was evaluated by intra-day and inter-day assays by performing replicate ($n = 6$) injections of six analytes as a mixed standard solution during a single day and by duplicating the experiments on three consecutive days. Variations of the peak area were taken as the measure of precision and expressed as percentage RSD. The overall intra-day and inter-day precisions were not more than 1.29% and 2.01%, respectively, as shown in Table 2.4. Stability of sample solutions stored at room temperature was investigated by replicate injections of the sample solution at 0, 2, 4, 8, 12 and 24 h. The RSD% of stability sample of the six analytes was ≤1.62%.

TABLE 2.4 Validation parameters for six reference analytes

	WITHANOSIDE IV	WITHAFERIN A	WITHANOSIDE V	WITHANONE	WITHANOLIDE A	WITHANOLIDE B
Regression equation	$y = 361.32x - 846.83$	$y = 1274.5x + 3894.2$	$y = 996.02x - 230.06$	$y = 1608.3x + 2366.6$	$y = 1594x - 1634.8$	$y = 8883.5x + 2181.2$
r^2	0.9996	0.9991	0.9990	0.9998	0.9989	0.9994
Linear range (ng mL^{-1})	10–500	0.5–250	1–100	0.5–250	0.5–100	0.5–50
LOD (ng mL^{-1})	2.11	0.06	0.18	0.04	0.02	0.03
LOQ (ng mL^{-1})	2.48	0.31	0.52	0.29	0.27	0.28
Precision RSD % (Intra-day, $n = 6$)	0.73	0.52	0.16	0.08	1.29	1.03
Precision RSD % (Inter-day, $n = 6$)	0.79	0.94	1.18	1.22	1.72	2.01
Stability RSD % ($n = 5$)	1.33	1.20	1.62	1.46	1.41	1.04
Recovery RSD %	2.45	2.04	1.14	1.39	1.07	2.02

Source: With permission from Chandra et al. 2016.

2.4 QUANTITATIVE ANALYSIS OF SIX MARKER COMPOUNDS

2.4.1 Five Varieties of *W. Somnifera* and Six Sodic Treatments

Six sodic treatments were carried out in five varieties of WS by manually altering different soil parameters such as pH, EC and ESP. The developed UPLC–MS/MS method was applied for the simultaneous determination of six marker compounds (withanolide A, withanolide B, withaferin A, withanone, withanoside IV and withanoside V) as shown in Figure 2.3 in samples of five varieties of WS (root, stem and leaf) extract under different sodic conditions. The contents calculated from the calibration curves are given in Table 2.5. These contents varied in varieties of the plant, different parts and in plants grown under different sodic conditions.

It is evident from Table 2.5 that withanolides are present in variable concentrations in different parts of the same plant and also in different plant types as reported earlier (Kaul et al. 2009). The contents of withanoside IV, withanoside V and withaferin A are the highest in the leaf followed by stem and the least in root in the variety 135 under T2 soil treatment conditions. In contrast, withanone and withanolide A contents are the highest in the roots of the variety 135 under T2 treatment conditions. Withanolide B content is not significant in any of the samples studied. Withaferin A is predominant in the leaves in all varieties except 108 under all the soil conditions studied. The stem contains the lowest content of total withanolides. T2 soil treatment condition (bulk density 1.36, pH 8.5, ESP 13% and EC 0.5 dSm^{-1}) was found to be the best soil conditions for highest content of withaferin A, withanolide A, withanolide B, withanone, withanoside IV and withanoside V. In root withanolide A (42300 µg/g) and withanone (39700 µg/g) were dominant in the variety 135 with T2 treatment condition. Similarly, maximum abundance of withanolide B (450 µg/g) was analysed in the root of variety 135 with T5 treatment condition at pH 9.3, ESP 30% and EC 0.8 dSm^{-1}). Leaf of variety 135 with T2 treatment condition contains the maximum abundance of withaferin A (58,500 µg/g), withanoside IV (14,600 µg/g) and withanoside IV (5950 µg/g). The stem contains the lowest content of total withanolides. It was observed that the variety 135 showed the highest abundance of major bioactive compounds in comparison to others, i.e., 101, 108, 118 and POS as shown in Table 2.5. In general, withanoside IV, withanoside V and withaferin A are

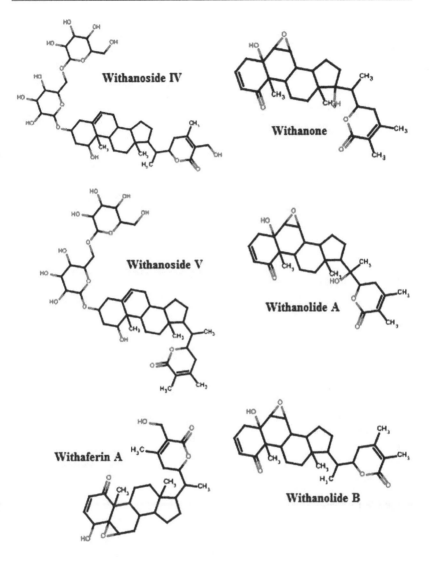

FIGURE 2.3 Structure of selected marker compounds of *W. somnifera* (with permission from Chandra et al. 2016).

found in highest quantities in leaf followed by stem and least in roots in all varieties under all soil treatment conditions. The contents of withanone and withanolide A were higher in the root than stem and leaf in all the varieties at T1 soil condition. However, variations were observed in other soil treatment conditions.

TABLE 2.5 Contents (μg/g) of the selected analytes in plants of *W. somnifera*

	WITHANOLIDE A			WITHANOLIDE B			WITHANONE			WITHAFERIN-A			WITHANOSIDE-IV			WITHANOSIDE-V		
	LEAF	STEM	ROOT	LEAF	STEM	ROOT	LEAF	STEM	ROOT	LEAF	STEM	ROOT	LEAF	STEM	ROOT	LEAF	STEM	ROOT
T_1-101	21000	5700	29600	140	30	30	21100	5950	27500	23500	5350	40	5900	3330	2430	2340	530	280
T_1-108	9950	4660	22000	60	10	70	9450	5000	21300	3200	840	50	4150	1360	540	510	320	90
T_1-118	9400	10500	29100	110	60	40	9500	10550	27150	22750	7850	0	6700	5750	600	1640	970	150
T_1-135	8500	2900	26350	100	10	60	8000	2950	25500	30550	3860	90	9650	3900	2140	2970	590	240
T_1-POS	3360	1270	24850	240	30	390	3150	1300	23250	54000	6550	2160	9000	3530	2820	2690	710	510
T_2-101	32000	5600	3580	60	nd	0	32450	5800	3430	42100	2230	nd	13350	3390	1920	4170	560	160
T_2-108	4970	2650	15550	150	nd	30	5100	2420	14300	12350	930	nd	3080	2420	540	2160	480	110
T_2-118	15150	1330	20050	180	110	20	15850	1430	19450	37950	2450	nd	10100	2860	430	3860	470	100
T_2-135	5800	9000	42300	160	150	250	5850	8550	39700	58500	21100	2160	14600	11600	1840	5950	2940	320
T_2-POS	16650	13050	nd	200	60	nd	15950	11700	nd	44450	10900	0	12050	4970	nd	4480	1570	nd
T_3-101	37400	8100	10350	70	30	60	34150	7750	9650	31200	5050	20	7650	5200	1910	2270	800	190
T_3-108	21400	5250	22300	180	60	nd	20950	5100	21600	11050	440	nd	3000	1680	610	600	270	120
T_3-118	24500	5800	nd	150	30	nd	26000	5900	nd	31400	9300	nd	4580	8550	nd	2350	1140	nd
T_3-135	5250	3880	nd	90	50	240	5650	3920	nd	45500	9550	nd	8550	9650	nd	2420	1250	230
T_3-POS	6450	6150	17850	150	60	60	6500	6450	16050	42000	12250	60	6200	5500	760	3910	1700	230
T_4-101	15300	5500	32750	90	60	100	15150	6300	31600	27300	3630	nd	7500	4790	1580	2750	670	260
T_4-108	6400	3280	14150	150	nd	40	6600	3300	12750	6550	20	nd	3460	2350	430	630	460	100
T_4-118	7550	5000	29800	140	70	160	6950	5300	30250	29650	7150	nd	5300	7850	300	2750	1010	130
T_4-135	520	2120	13350	80	30	10	590	2190	13400	38550	14050	nd	4450	5300	310	2340	1250	160
T_4-POS	10700	5450	680	120	20	60	9700	5300	620	45950	6550	nd	5800	4350	270	2410	770	110
T_5-101	21050	17100	22900	120	140	30	19650	17750	20950	23500	11400	nd	4310	9400	330	1100	1440	120
T_5-108	6750	6650	8000	40	20	180	6700	6550	7450	3550	1410	nd	4470	2610	290	490	540	90
T_5-118	19050	4080	41950	220	50	450	18000	4080	36900	39350	5150	80	7400	5100	340	3210	740	140
T_5-135	6700	8900	30700	110	100	210	6900	9100	26750	30500	9600	nd	4350	6550	390	2850	1450	130
T_5-POS	8850	4260	35050	90	10	20	8650	4310	32850	42050	5250	80	6200	4180	630	2800	1570	280
T_6-101	14100	5700	14100	170	70	50	16150	5550	14200	35100	6500	nd	7800	4780	750	3700	1000	140
T_6-108	9200	7650	7150	110	80	30	9750	6650	6800	11400	3550	nd	3180	3020	590	910	750	80
T_6-118	18400	16650	25800	210	330	130	17650	16100	22400	27300	10550	nd	6300	8550	1260	2730	1760	170
T_6-135	16000	5350	23300	180	50	80	16650	5500	22100	41750	8200	310	4590	3630	1250	1750	740	180
T_6-POS	14900	3670	27950	150	40	nd	12900	3860	27200	53500	7550	nd	7150	3670	310	4190	1050	130

Source: With permission from Chandra et al. 2016.
nd: not detected

2.4.2 Herbal Formulations

The six marker compounds (withanolide A, withanolide B, withaferin A, withanone, withanoside IV and withanoside V) were also determined in 26 different marketed formulations including tablets and capsules of various herbal formulation manufactures obtained from the local market. The method proved to be effective and reliable in estimating the selected marker contents summarized in Table 2.6. The contents of withanolide A, withanolide B and withanone were highest in formulation F-18 (375 µg/g, 49 µg/g and 360 µg/g, respectively). Similarly, maximum contents of withaferin A, withanoside IV and withanoside V were observed in formulation F-19 (1905 µg/g, 845 µg/g and 500 µg/g, respectively). In a few formulations, these compounds were found in moderate amount, whereas in others, such as F-15 and F-16, these were found below the detection limit. As shown in Table 2.6 the concentration of each analyte varied greatly among the different formulations. This could be due to different growing conditions and climate affecting the phytochemical content of WS and differences in processing of crude herbs.

2.5 QUALITY ASSESSMENT OF HERBAL FORMULATIONS BY HCA AND PCA

2.5.1 Hierarchical Clustering Analysis

Multivariate analysis (HCA and PCA) was applied for the quality assessment of herbal formulations. As shown in the dendogram of herbal formulations in Figure 2.4, the HCA of the contents of six marker compounds of 26 herbal formulations revealed that there is a profound similarity of the quantities of six markers of WS in the majority (20) of formulations, namely F1–F8, F12–F16 and F20–F26. These formulations appear in a single cluster. F9 and F11 are in close similarity to the first cluster of 20 formulations. F17 and F10 are different due to the comparatively higher quantities of withanolides. Similarly, F18 and F19 are entirely different from the rest of formulations due to the presence of the highest and next highest quantities of total withanolides. HCA was also performed on withanolide contents of root, stem and leaf of WS as shown in Figure 2.5. It is probably the first reporting of grouping of WS varieties. The cluster analysis of stem identifies S9 as outstanding variety. The distribution of chemicals in S9 is substantially different from the other varieties of WS. The remaining varieties are distributed into four groups. The segmentation

TABLE 2.6   Content (μg/g) of the selected analytes in different polyherbal marketed formulation of *W. somnifera*

SAMPLE CODE	W. SOMNIFERA COMPOSITION	WITHANOLIDE A	WITHANOLIDE B	WITHANONE	WITHAFERIN A	WITHANOSIDE IV	WITHANOSIDE V	TOTAL
F-1	30 mg	25.5	3.075	28.75	nd	42	21.775	121.10
F-2	25 mg	13.475	0.3275	13.1	nd	41.5	20.825	89.23
F-3	0.25 mg	nd	Nd	nd	nd	9.325	5.475	14.80
F-4	15 mg	14.625	2.775	13.475	40.75	44.5	21.975	138.10
F-5	4.26 g	0.05	Nd	0.275	0.575	10.5	6.125	17.53
F-6	100 mg	23.85	2.1025	20.25	7.4	9.775	7.95	71.33
F-7	1 g	3.725	Nd	6.525	nd	34.75	14.675	59.68
F-8	40 mg	6.925	0.32	7.15	nd	33.75	20.175	68.32
F-9	25 mg	52.75	7.25	47.5	109.5	43.25	28.75	289.00
F-10	100 g	22.4	Nd	21.325	547.5	224.5	155.5	971.23
F-11	70 mg	41.5	5.05	45.25	113.5	62.25	30.25	297.80
F-12	200 mg	nd	Nd	nd	nd	nd	4.15	4.15
F-13	50 mg	30	4.025	31.5	49.25	34.25	24.775	173.80
F-14	15 mg	23.1	3.35	25.5	65.75	48.25	27.5	193.45
F-15	218.75 mg	nd	0.935	nd	nd	nd	5.825	6.76
F-16	25 mg	nd	0.3875	0.71	nd	11	7.9	20.00
F-17	50 mg	4.3	Nd	5.35	177	115.25	85.5	387.40
F-18	300 mg	375	49	360	212.75	562.5	181.5	1740.75
F-19	250 mg	233.75	2.775	209.5	1905	845	500	3696.03
F-20	78 mg	9.875	0.7875	11.925	33.5	35	20.125	111.21
F-21	30 mg	6.325	0.98	7.375	7.2	25.25	13.25	60.38
F-22	45 mg	2.525	Nd	nd	0.175	12.775	8.05	23.53
F-23	81 mg	11.65	1.185	12.15	3.3	22.7	15.05	66.04
F-24	71 mg	14.7	0.3925	14.925	nd	68.5	32.75	131.27
F-25	20 mg	nd	Nd	nd	nd	5.825	4.05	9.88
F-26	130 mg	22.55	2.525	21.8	61.25	34.5	22.875	165.50

Source: With permission from Chandra et al. 2016.
nd: not detected

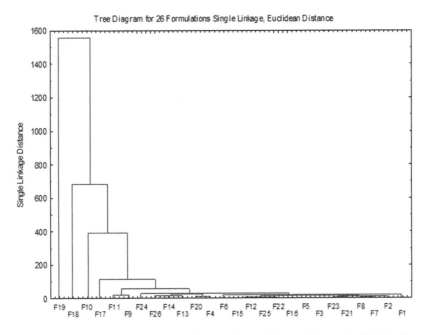

FIGURE 2.4 Quality assessment of 26 polyherbal formulations by HCA (with permission from Chandra et al. 2016).

of varieties helps to reveal similar varieties. Homogeneous groups were also observed in root and leaf.

2.5.2 Principal Component Analysis

To analyze, classify and reduce the dimensionality of numerical datasets in a multivariate problem, PCA was used as an unsupervised pattern recognition method. PCA was also carried out to compare and evaluate the quality of 26 different formulations based on the characteristics of six investigated compounds. PCA analysis showed that the whole information of WS is covered by two principal components. The PC1 shares 76.85% and PC2 shares 22.76% variation of data matrix as shown in Figure 2.6. PC plot of WS parameters shows equal division of parameters due to the sign of loadings of PC2. Compounds withanoside IV, withaferin A and withanoside V were in one group and withanone, withanolide A and withanolide B were in another group. It is clearly evident from the biplot of WS UPLC–MS/MS data that formulations F1–F8, F12–F16 and F20–F26 were falling in one group, while F9 and F11 were in second group and the remaining formulations F10, F17, F18 and

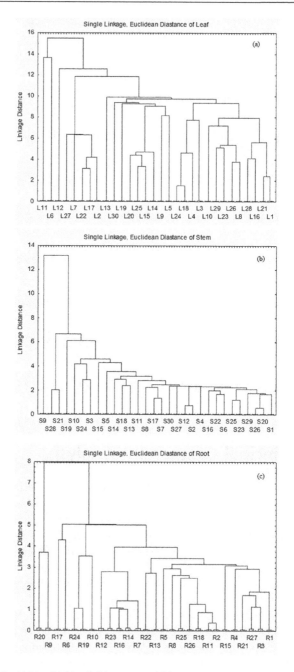

FIGURE 2.5 HCA of (a) leaf, (b) stem and (c) root.

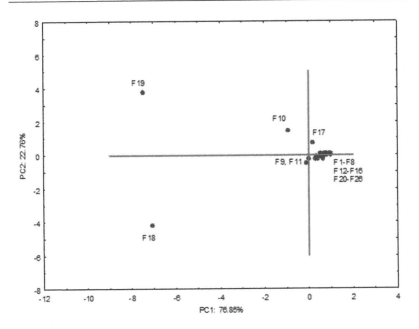

FIGURE 2.6 Quality assessment of 26 polyherbal formulations by PCA, score plot of 26 polyherbal formulations with respect to six reference analytes (with permission from Chandra et al. 2016).

F19 were distinct from each other. The two groups have similarity in the quantity of six marker compounds. Quantitative scores of formulation F19 were dominated by the PC2 loadings of withanoside IV, withaferin A and withanoside V while that of formulation F18 were influenced by the negative PC1 and PC2 loadings of withanone, withanolide A and withanolide B. These results are in agreement with the earlier reported phytochemical variability of several mono and polyherbal formulations of Withania (Sangwan et al. 2004).

2.6 CONCLUSION

A rapid and accurate UPLC-ESI-QqQ$_{LIT}$-MS/MS method was developed for the quantitative analysis of selected withanolides in WS. The simultaneous quantitative analysis of six withanolides in five varieties of WS and in different plant parts (root, stem and leaf) of WS was accomplished. This method is also applicable to assess the quality of commercial formulated products containing WS bioactive compounds. It not only allows the direct, rapid and accurate determination of withanolides, but also fulfills all criteria of a validated method with respect to precision, repeatability and accuracy as per ICH guidelines. Results indicated that WS variety NMITLI-135 grown in sodic soil at conditions of pH 8.5, ESP-13 and EC 0.5 dSm^{-1} had the maximum content of withanolides. Multiple reaction monitoring is convenient for complex multi-component analytical determination of various herbal formulations. The developed method was found to be suitable for routine quality assessment and control of raw materials and finished products.

References

1. Abdel-Wahhab, K. G., H. H. Mourad, F. A. Mannaa, F. A. Morsy, L. K. Hassan and R. F. Taher. "Role of Ashwagandha methanolic extract in the regulation of thyroid profile in hypothyroidism modeled rats." *Molecular Biology Reports* 46, no. 4 (2019): 3637–3649.
2. Abou-Douh, A. M. "New withanolides and other constituents from the fruit of Withania somnifera." *Archiv der Pharmazie (Weinheim)* 335, no. 6 (2002): 267–276.
3. Abraham, A., I. Kirson, E. Glotter and D. Lavie. "A chemotaxonomic study of Withania somnifera (L.) Dunal." *Phytochemistry* 7 (1968): 957–962.
4. Achini, D. K. N., R. Aku, J. Krutika and S. Gaurav. "Review on ergogenic effect of Withania somnifera (L.) Dunal." *International Ayurvedic Medical Journal* 2020 (2020): 4219–4228. doi.org/10.46607/iamj0807332020
5. Adaikkappan, P., M. Kannapiran and A. Anthonisamy. "Anti-mycobacterial activity of Withania somnifera and Pueraria tuberosa against Mycobacterium tuberculosis H37Rv." *Journal of Academia and Industrial Research* 1, no. 4 (2012): 153–156.
6. Ahmad, M. and N. J. Dar, "Withania somnifera: Ethnobotany, pharmacology, and therapeutic functions in sustained energy for enhanced human functions and activity." In D. Bagchi (ed.) *Sustained Energy for Enhanced Human Functions and Activity*, London: Academic Press (2017): 137–154.
7. Ahmad, M. K., A. A. Mahdi, K. K. Shukla, et al. "Withania somnifera improves semen quality by regulating reproductive hormone levels and oxidative stress in seminal plasma of infertile males." *Fertility and Sterility* 94, no. 3 (2010): 989–96.
8. Ahmad, M. K., R. Singh, S. N. Shankhwar, V. Singh and D. Dalela." Withania somnifera improves semen quality in stress-related male fertility." *Evidence-Based Complementary and Alternative Medicine* (2011): Article ID 576962. doi:10.1093/ecam/nep138
9. Ahmed, M. E., H. Javed, M. M. Khan, et al. "Attenuation of oxidative damage-associated cognitive decline by Withania somnifera in rat model of streptozotocin-induced cognitive impairment." *Protoplasma* 250, no. 5 (2013): 1067–1078.
10. Akhoon, B. A., L. Rathor and R. Pandey. "Withanolide A extends the lifespan in human EGFR-driven cancerous Caenorhabditis elegans." *Experimental Gerontology* 104 (2018): 113–117.
11. Alam, M. K., M. O. Hoq and M. S. Uddin. "Therapeutic use of Withania somnifera." *Asian Journal of Medical and Biological Research* 2, no. 2 (2016): 148–155.
12. Alam, N., M. Hossain, M. I. Khalil, M. Moniruzzaman, S. A. Sulaiman and S. H. Gan. "High catechin concentrations detected in Withania somnifera (Ashwagandha) by high performance liquid chromatography analysis." *BMC Complementary and Alternative Medicine* 11 (2011): 65.

13. Ali, A. S., S. H., Bashir. and K. A. Abdelshafeek. "Isolation, identification of some chemical constituents and antimicrobial activity of different extracts from Withania somnifera growing at Albaha region, KSA." *Biomedical & Pharmacology Journal* 13, no. 2 (2020): 635–644.

14. Ali, N. W., S. Abouzid, A. Nasib, S. Khan, J. Qureshi and M. I. Choudhary. "RP-HPLC analysis of withanolides in the flowers, leaves, and roots of Withania somnifera." *Acta Chromatographica* 22, no. 3 (2010): 473–480.

15. Alzoubi, K. H., A. S. Al Hilo, Q. A. Al-Balas, K. El-Salem, T. El-Elimat and F. Q. Alali. "Withania somnifera root powder protects against post-traumatic stress disorder-induced memory impairment." *Molecular Biology Reports* 46, no. 5 (2019): 4709–4715.

16. Andallu, B. and B. Radhika. "Hypoglycemic, diuretic and hypocholesterolemic effect of winter cherry (Withania somnifera) root." *Indian Journal of Experimental Biology* 38, no. 6 (2000): 607–609.

17. Andrade, C., A. Aswath, S. K. Chaturvedi, M. Srinivasa and R. Raguram. "A double-blind, placebo-controlled evaluation of the anxiolytic efficacy of an ethanolic extract of Withania somnifera." *Indian Journal of Psychiatry* 42, no. 3 (2000): 295–301.

18. Anjaneyulu, A. S. R. and D. S. Rao. "New withanolides from the roots of Withania somnifera." *Indian Journal of Chemistry* 36B (1997): 424–433.

19. Anonymous. "Monograph. Withania somnifera." *Alternative Medicine Review* 9, no. 2 (2004): 211–214.

20. Antony, B., A. P. A. Aravind, M. Benny, N. K. Gupta, B. Joseph and A. Sebastian. "Bioactivity guided fractionation and purification of anti-depressant molecule from Ashwagandha (Withania somnifera)." *Current Bioactive Compounds* 16, no. 5 (2020): 681–686.

21. Anwer, T., M. Sharma, K. K. Pillai and G. Khan. "Protective effect of Withania somnifera against oxidative stress and pancreatic beta-cell damage in type 2 diabetic rats." *Acta Poloniae Pharmaceutica* 69, no. 6 (2012): 1095–1101.

22. Anwer, T., M. Sharma, K. K. Pillai and M. Iqbal. "Effect of Withania somnifera on insulin sensitivity in non-insulin-dependent diabetes mellitus rats." *Basic & Clinical Pharmacology & Toxicology* 102, no. 6 (2008): 498–503.

23. Archana, R. and A. Namasivayam. "Antistressor effect of Withania somnifera." *Journal of Ethnopharmacology* 64, no. 1 (1999): 91–93.

24. Atal, C. K., O. P. Gupta, K. Raghunanthan and K. L. Dhar. *Pharmacognosy and Phytochemistry of Withania Somnifera (Linn.) Dunal (Ashwagandha)*, New Delhi: Central Council for Research in Indian Medicine and Homoeopathy (1975): 47–53.

25. Azgomi, R. N. D., A. Zomorrodi, H. Nazemyieh, et al. "Effects of Withania somnifera on reproductive system: As review of the available evidence." *BioMed Research International* 2018 (2018): Article ID 4076430.

26. Baek, S. C., S. Lee, S. Kim, et al. "Withaninsams A and B: Phenylpropanoid esters from the roots of Indian Ginseng (Withania somnifera)." *Plants (Basel)* 8, no. 12 (2019): 527.

27. Bala, S., R. Govindrajan, A. K. S. Rawat and S. Mahrotra. "HPLC analysis of withaferin A in Withania somnifera (L.) Dunal." *Indian Journal of Pharmaceutical Sciences* 66 (2004): 236–238.

28. Balekundri, A. and V. Mannur. "Quality control of the traditional herbs and herbal products: A review." *Future Journal of Pharmaceutical Sciences* 6 (2020): 67.

29. Bano, A., N. Sharma, H. S. Dhaliwal and V. Sharma. "A systematic and comprehensive review on Withania somnifera (L.) Dunal—An Indian Ginseng." *British Journal of Pharmaceutical Research* 7, no. 2 (2015): 63–75.

30. Bashir, H. S., A. M. Mohammed, A. S. Magsoud and A. M. Shaoub. "Isolation of three flavonoids from Withania somnifera leaves (Solanaceae) and their antimicrobial activities." *Journal of Forest Products & Industries* 2, no. 5 (2013): 39–45.

31. Bassareo, V., G. Talani, R. Frau, et al. "Inhibition of morphine- and ethanol-mediated stimulation of mesolimbic dopamine neurons by Withania somnifera." *Frontiers in Neuroscience* 13 (2019): 545. doi: 10.3389/fnins.2019.00545

32. Bessalle, R. and D. Lavie. "Semi-quantitative reverse-phase high performance liquid chromatographic analysis of Withania somnifera chemotype III." *Journal of Chromatography* 389 (1987): 195–210.

33. Bharti, S. K., A. Bhatia, S. K. Tewari, O. P. Sidhu and R. Roy. "Application of HR-MAS NMR spectroscopy for studying chemotype variations of Withania somnifera (L.) Dunal." *Magnetic Resonance in Chemistry* 49 (2011): 659–667.

34. Bhatia, A., S. K. Kharti, S. K. Rewari, O. P. Sidhu and R. Roy. "Metabolic profiling for studying chemotype variations in Withania somnifera (L.) Dunal fruits using GC-MS and NMR spectroscopy." *Phytochemistry* 93 (2013): 105–115.

35. Bhattacharya, A., M. Ramanathan, S. Ghosal and S. K. Bhattacharya. "Effect of Withania somnifera glycowithanolides on iron-induced hepatotoxicity in rats." *Phytotherapy Research* 17, no. 7 (2000a): 568–570.

36. Bhattacharya, S. K., A. Bhattacharya, K. Sairam and S. Ghosal. "Anxiolytic-antidepressant activity of Withania somnifera glycowithanolides: An experimental study." *Phytomedicine* 7, no. 6 (2000b): 463–469.

37. Bhattacharya, S. K. and A. V. Muruganandam. "Adaptogenic activity of Withania somnifera: An experimental study using a rat model of chronic stress." *Pharmacology Biochemistry and Behavior* 75, no. 3 (2003): 547–555.

38. Bhattacharya, S. K., K. S. Satyan and S. Ghosal. "Antioxidant activity of glycowithanolides from Withania somnifera." *Indian Journal of Experimental Biology* 35, no. 3 (1997): 236–239.

39. Bhattacharya, S. K., R. K. Goel, R. Kaur and S. Ghosal. "Anti-stress activity of sitoindosides VII and VIII, new acylsterylglucosides from Withania somnifera." *Phytotherapy Research* 1, no. 1 (1987): 32–37.

40. Birla, H., C. Keswani, S. N. Rai, et al. "Neuroprotective effects of Withania somnifera in BPA induced-cognitive dysfunction and oxidative stress in mice." *Behavioral and Brain Functions* 15, no. 1 (2019): 9. doi: 10.1186/s12993-019-0160-4

41. Biswal, B. M., S. A. Sulaiman, H. C. Ismail, H. Zakaria and K. I. Musa. "Effect of Withania somnifera (Ashwagandha) on the development of chemotherapy-induced fatigue and quality of life in breast cancer patients." *Integrative Cancer Therapies* 12, no. 4 (2013): 312–322.

42. Björnsson, H. K., E. S. Björnsson, B. Avula, et al. "Ashwagandha-induced liver injury: A case series from Iceland and the US drug-induced liver injury network." *Liver International* 40, no. 4 (2020): 825–829.

43. Bolleddula, J., W. Fitch, S. K. Vareed and M. G. Nair. "Identification of metabolites in Withania somnifera fruits by liquid chromatography and high resolution mass spectrometry." *Rapid Communications in Mass Spectrometry* 26, no. 11 (2012): 1277–1290.

44. Bone, K. *Clinical Applications of Ayurvedic and Chinese Herbs: Monographs for the Western Herbal Practitioner*, Queensland, Australia: Phytotherapy Press (1996): 137–141.

45. Bonilla, D. A., Y. Moreno, C. Gho, et al. "Effect of Ashwagandha (Withania somnifera) on physical performance: Systematic review and Bayesian meta-analysis." *Journal of Functional Morphology and Kinesiology* 6 (2021): 20. https://doi.org/10.3390/jfmk6010020

46. Budhiraja, R. D., P. Krishnan and S. Sudhir. "Biological activity of withanolides." *Journal of Scientific and Industrial Research* 59 (2000): 904–911.

47. Bungau, S., C. M. Vesa, A. Abid, et al. Withaferin A—A promising phytochemical compound with multiple results in dermatological diseases. *Molecules* 26 (2021): 2407. doi.org/10.3390/molecules26092407

48. Caputi, F. F., E. Acquas, S. Kasture, S. Ruiu, S. Candeletti and P. Romualdi. "The standardized Withania somnifera Dunal root extract alters basal and morphine-induced opioid receptor Gene expression changes in neuroblastoma cells." *BMC Complementary and Alternative Medicine* 18 (2018): 9. doi: 10.1186/s12906-017-2065-9

49. Chadha, Y. R. *The Wealth of India*, Vol. X, New Delhi: Publications and Information Directorate, CSIR (1976): 582.

50. Chandra, P., R. Pandey, M. Srivastva and B. Kumar. "Quality control assessment of polyherbal formulation based on a quantitative determination multi-marker approach by ultra high performance liquid chromatography with tandem mass spectrometry using polarity switching combined with multivariate analysis." *Journal of Separation Science* 38 (2015): 3183–3191.

51. Chandra, P., R. Kannujia, A. Saxena, et al. "Quantitative determination of multi markers in five varieties of Withania somnifera using ultra-high performance liquid chromatography with hybrid triple quadrupole linear ion trap mass spectrometer combined with multivariate analysis: Application to pharmaceutical dosage forms." *Journal of Pharmaceutical and Biomedical Analysis* 129 (2016): 419–426.

52. Chandrasekaran, S., J. Veronica, S. Sundar and R. Maurya. "Alcoholic fractions F5 and F6 from Withania somnifera leaves show a potent antileishmanial and immunomodulatory activities to control experimental visceral leishmaniasis." *Frontiers in Medicine (Lausanne)* 4 (2017): 55.

53. Chandrasekhar, K., J. Kapoor and S. Anishetty. "A prospective, randomized, double-blind, placebo-controlled study of safety and efficacy of a high-concentration full spectrum extract of Ashwagandha root in reducing stress and anxiety in adults." *Indian Journal of Psychology and Medicine* 34, no. 3 (2012): 255–262.

54. Chatterjee, S., S. Srivastava, A. Khalid, et al. "Comprehensive metabolic fingerprinting of Withania somnifera leaf and root extracts." *Phytochemistry* 71, no. 10 (2010): 1085–1094.

55. Chauhan, S., A. Joshi, R. Jain and D. Jain. "Estimation of withanolide A in diverse genotypes of Ashwagandha/Withania somnifera (L.) Dunal." *Indian Journal of Experimental Biology* 57, no. 3 (2019): 212–217.

56. Chaurasiya, N. D., R. S. Sangwan, L. N. Misra, R. Tuli and N. S. Sangwan. "Metabolic clustering of a core collection of Indian ginseng (Withania somnifera) through DNA, isoenzymes, polypeptide and withanolide profile diversity." *Fitoterapia* 80 (2009): 496–505.

57. Chaurasiya, N. D., G. C. Uniyal, P. Lal, L. Misra, N. S. Sangwan, R. Tuli and R. S. Sangwan. "Analysis of withanolides in root and leaf of Withania somnifera by HPLC with photodiode array and evaporative light scattering detection." *Phytochemical Analysis* 19, no. 2 (2008): 148–154.

58. Chen, L. X., H. He and F. Qiu. "Natural withanolides: An overview." *Natural Products Reports* 28, no. 4 (2011): 705–740.

59. Chengappa, K. N., C. R. Bowie, P. J. Schlicht, D. Fleet, J. S. Brar and R. Jindal. "Randomized placebo-controlled adjunctive study of an extract of Withania somnifera for cognitive dysfunction in bipolar disorder." *Journal of Clinical Psychiatry* 74, no. 11 (2013): 1076–1083.

60. Choudhary, M. I., S. Yousuf and Atta-ur-Rahman. "Withanolides: Chemistry and Antitumor Activity." In K. Ramawat and J. M. Mérillon (eds.) *Natural Products*, Heidelberg: Springer (2013).

61. Choudhary, B., A. Shetty and D. G. Langade. "Efficacy of Ashwagandha (Withania somnifera [L.] Dunal) in improving cardiorespiratory endurance in healthy athletic adults." *Ayu* 36, no. 1 (2015): 63–68.

62. Choudhary, D., S. Bhattacharyya and K. Joshi. "Body weight management in adults under chronic stress through treatment with Ashwagandha root extract a double-blind, randomized, placebo-controlled trial." *Journal of Evidence Based Complementary and Alternative Medicine* 22, no. 1 (2017b): 96–106.

63. Choudhary, D., S. Bhattacharyya and S. Bose. "Efficacy and safety of Ashwagandha [Withania somnifera (L.) Dunal] root extract in improving memory and cognitive functions." *Journal of Dietary Supplements* 16, no. 6 (2017a): 599–612.

64. Choudhary, M. I., S. Yousuf, S. A. Nawaz and S. Ahmed. "Cholinesterase inhibiting withanolides from Withania somnifera." *Chemical and Pharmaceutical Bulletin* 52, no. 11 (2004): 1358–1361.

65. Cooley, K., O. Szczurko, D. Perri, et al. "Naturopathic care for anxiety: A randomized controlled trial ISRCTN78958974." *PLoS One* 4, no. 8 (2009): e6628.

66. Dagar, J. C. and O. S. Tomar. "Cultivation of medicinal isabgol (Planta ocata) in alkali soils in semiarid regions of Northern India." *Land Degradation and Development* 17 (2006): 275–283.

67. Dar, N. J. and M. Ahmad. "Neurodegenerative diseases and Withania somnifera (L.): An update." *Journal of Ethnopharmacology* 256 (2020): 112769. doi:10.1016/j.jep.2020.112769

68. Dar, N. J., A. Hamid and M. Ahmad. "Pharmacologic overview of Withania somnifera, the Indian ginseng." *Cellular and Molecular Life Sciences* 72, no. 23 (2015): 4445–4460.

69. Dar, P. A., L. R. Singh, M. A. Kamal and T. A. Dar. "Unique medicinal properties of Withania somnifera: Phytochemical constituents and protein component." *Current Pharmaceutical Design* 22, no. 5 (2016): 535–540.

70. Datta, A. K., A. Das, A. Bhattacharya, S. Mukherjee and B. K. Ghosh. "An overview of Withania somnifera (L.) Dunal—The Indian ginseng." *Medicinal and Aromatic Plant Science and Biotechnology* 5, no. 1 (2011): 1–15.

71. Davis, L. and G. Kuttan. "Immunomodulatory activity of Withania somnifera." *Journal of Ethnopharmacology* 71, no. 1–2 (2000): 193–200.

72. Debnath, P. K., J. Chattopadhyay, A. Mitra, et al. "Adjunct therapy of Ayurvedic medicine with anti tubercular drugs on the therapeutic management of pulmonary tuberculosis." *Journal of Ayurveda and Integrative Medicine* 3, no. 3 (2012): 141–149.

73. Deshpande, A., N. Irani, R. Balkrishnan and I. R. Benny. "A randomized double blind, placebo controlled study to evaluate the effects of Ashwagandha (Withania somnifera) extract on sleep quality in healthy adults." *Sleep Medicine* 72 (2020): 28–36.

74. Dey, A., S. S. Chatterjee and V. Kumar. "Analgesic activity of a Withania somnifera extract in stressed mice." *Oriental Pharmacy and Experimental Medicine* 16 (2016): 295–302.

75. Dhalla, N. S., M. S. Sastry and C. L. Malhotra. "Chemical studies of the leaves of Withania somnifera." *Journal of Pharmaceutical Sciences* 50, no. 10 (1961): 876–877.

76. Dhar, R. S., S. B. Gupta, P. P. Singh, et al. "Identification and characterization of protein composition in Withania somnifera—An Indian ginseng." *Journal of Plant Biochemistry and Biotechnology* 21 (2012): 77–87.

77. Dhar, N., S. Rana, W. W. Bhat, et al. "Dynamics of withanolide biosynthesis in relation to temporal expression pattern of metabolic genes in Withania somnifera (L.) Dunal: A comparative study in two morpho-chemovariants." *Molecular Biology Reports* 40 (2013): 7007–7016.

78. Dhar, R. S., V. Verma, K. A. Suri, et al. "Phytochemical and genetic analysis in selected chemotypes of Withania somnifera." *Phytochemistry* 67 (2006): 2269–2276. doi: 10.1016/j.phytochem.2006.07.014

79. Dikasso, D., E. Makonnen, A. Debella, et al. "Anti-malarial activity of Withania somnifera L. Dunal extracts in mice." *Ethiopian Medical Journal* 44, no. 3 (2006): 279–285.

80. Dongre, S., D. Langade and S. Bhattacharyya. "Efficacy and safety of Ashwagandha (Withania somnifera) root extract in improving sexual function in women: A pilot study." *Biomedical Research International* 2015 (2015): 284154.

81. Durg, S., S. Bavage and S. B. Shivaram. "Withania somnifera (Indian ginseng) in diabetes mellitus: A systematic review and meta-analysis of scientific evidence from experimental research to clinical application." *Phytotherapy Research* 34, no. 5 (2020): 1041–1059.

82. Dutta, R., R. Khalil, R. Green, S. S. Mohapatra and S. Mohapatra. "Withania somnifera (Ashwagandha) and withaferin A: Potential in integrative oncology." *International Journal of Molecular Sciences* 20, no. 21 (2019): 5310.

83. El-Hefny, M., M. Z. M. Salem, S. I. Behiry and H. M. Ali. "The potential antibacterial and antifungal activities of wood treated with Withania somnifera fruit extract, and the phenolic, caffeine, and flavonoid composition of the extract according to HPLC." *Processes* 8, no. 1 (2020): 113.

84. Facciola, S. *Cornucopia–A Source Book of Edible Plants*, Vista, California: Kampong Publications (1990).

85. Farooqui, A. A., T. Farooqui, A. Madan, J. H-J. Ong and W-Y. Ong. "Ayurvedic medicine for the treatment of dementia: Mechanistic aspects." *Evidence-Based Complementary and Alternative Medicine* 2018 (2018): 2481076.

86. Filipiak-Szok, A., M. Kurzawa, E. Szlyk, M. Twaruzek, A. Blajet-Kosicka and J. Grajewski. "Determination of mycotoxins, alkaloids, phytochemicals, antioxidants and cytotoxicity in Asiatic ginseng (Ashwagandha, Dong quai, Panax ginseng)." *Chemical Papers- Slovak Academy of Sciences* 71 (2017): 1073–1082.

87. Forman, M. and N. A. Kerna. "Merging Ayurvedic Ashwagandha with traditional Chinese medicine part 1. Foundation in Ashwagandha: Physiological effects, clinical efficacy, and properties." *Current Research in Complementary and Alternative Medicine*. CRCAM-133. 2018, no. 1 (2018): 1–6. DOI:10.29011/2577-2201/100033

88. Frawley, D. and V. Lad *The Yoga of Herbs: An Ayurvedic Guide to Herbal Medicine*, 4th ed. New Delhi: Motilal Banarsidass Publishing House (2016).

89. Funde, S. G. "Analysis of active pharmaceutical ingredients and antioxidant potential of Ayurvedic medicinal plants." *Specialty Journal of Medical Research And Health Science* 4, no. 4 (2019): 23–34.

90. Gajarmal, A. A., M. B. Shende and D. S. Chothe. "Antistress activity of Ashwagandha (Withania somnifera Dunal." *International Ayurvedic Medical Journal* 2, no. 3 (2014): 387–393.

91. Gajbhiye, N. A., J. Makasana and S. Kumar. "Accumulation of three important bioactive compounds in different plant parts of Withania somnifera and its determination by the LC–ESI-MS-MS (MRM) method." *Journal of Chromatographic Science* 53, no. 10 (2015): 1749–1756.

92. Gannon, J. M., J. Brar, A. Rai and K. N. R. Chengappa. Effects of a standardized extract of Withania somnifera (Ashwagandha) on depression and anxiety symptoms in persons with schizophrenia participating in a randomized, placebo-controlled clinical trial. *Annals of Clinical Psychiatry* 31, no. 2 (2019): 123–129.

93. Ganzera, M., M. I. Choudhary and I. A. Khan. "Quantitative HPLC analysis of withanolides in Withania somnifera." *Fitoterapia* 74, no. 1–2 (2003): 68–76.

94. Gao, S., H. Li, X. Q. Zhou, et al. "Withaferin A attenuates lipopolysaccharide-induced acute lung injury in neonatal rats." *Cellular and Molecular Biology (Noisy-le-grand)* 61, no. 3 (2015): 102–106.

95. Gavande, K., K. Jain, B. Jain and R. Mehta. "Comprehensive report on phytochemistry and pharmacological prominence of Withania somnifera." *UK Journal of Pharmaceutical and Biosciences* 3, no. 2 (2015): 15–23.

96. Geetha, A., N. G. Wasnik and K. Kalaiselvi. "HPLC analysis of different parts of Withania somnifera." *Natural Products: An Indian Journal* 6, no. 3 (2010): 125–127.

97. Ghosal, S., J. Lal and R. Srivastava et al. "Immunomodulatory and CNS effects of sitoindosides IX and X, two new glycowithanolides from Withania somnifera." *Phytotherapy Research* 3, no. 5 (1989): 201–206.

98. Girish, K. S., K. D. Machiah, S. Ushanandini, et al. "Antimicrobial properties of a non-toxic glycoprotein (WSG) from Withania somnifera (Ashwagandha)." *Journal of Basic Microbiology* 46, no. 5 (2006): 365–374.

99. Girme, A., G. Saste, S. Pawar, et al. "Investigating 11 withanosides and withanolides by UHPLC–PDA and mass fragmentation studies from Ashwagandha (Withania somnifera)." *ACS Omega* 5, no. 43 (2020): 27933–27943.

100. Goraya, G. S. and D. K. Ved. *Medicinal Plants in India: An Assessment of Their Demand and Supply*, Dehradun: National Medicinal Plants Board and Indian Council of Forestry Research & Education (2017).

101. Govindappa, P. K., V. Gautam, S. M. Tripathi, Y. P. Sahni and H. L. Raghavendra. "Effect of Withania somnifera on gentamicin induced renal lesions in rats." *Revista Brasileira de Farmacognosia* 29, no. 2 (2019): 234–240.

102. Grover, A., S. P. Katiyar, J. Jeyakanthan, V. K. Dubey and D. Sundar. "Blocking protein kinase C signaling pathway: Mechanistic insights into the anti-leishmanial activity of prospective herbal drugs from Withania somnifera." *BMC Genomics* 13, no. S7 (2012): S20.

103. Gupta, A. and S. Singh. "Evaluation of anti-inflammatory effect of Withania somnifera root on collagen-induced arthritis in rats." *Pharmaceutical Biology* 52, no. 3 (2014): 308–320.

104. Gupta, G. L. and A. C. Rana. "Withania somnifera (Ashwagandha): A review." *Pharmacognosy Reviews* 1, no. 1 (2007): 129–136.

105. Gupta, M. and G. Kaur. "Withania somnifera (L.) Dunal ameliorates neuro-degeneration and cognitive impairments associated with systemic inflammation." *BMC Complementary and Alternative Medicine* 19, no. 1 (2019): 217. doi. org/10.1186/s12906-019-2635-0

106. Gupta, Y. K., S. S. Sharma, K. Rai, et al. "Reversal of paclitaxel induced neutropenia by Withania somnifera in mice." *Indian Journal of Physiology and Pharmacology* 45, no. 2 (2001): 253–257.

107. Halder, T. and B. Ghosh. "Phytochemical and pharmacological activity of Withania somnifera (L.) Dunal." *International Journal of Economic Plants* 2, no. 4 (2015): 192–196.

108. Hameed, A. and N. Akhtar. "Comparative chemical investigation and evaluation of antioxidant and tyrosinase inhibitory effects of Withania somnifera (L.) Dunal and Solanum nigrum (L.) berries." *Acta Pharmaceutica* 68, no. 1 (2018): 47–60.

109. Husain, G. M., D. Mishra, P. N. Singh, C. V. Rao and V. Kumar. "Ethnopharmacological review of native traditional medicinal plants for brain disorders." *Pharmacognosy Review* 1, no. 1 (2007): 19–29.

110. Ismail, S. K. "Quantitative evolution of withanolides content of Egyptian Withania somnifera (L.) roots." *Al-Azhar Journal of Pharmaceutical Sciences* 47, no. 1 (2013): 95–104.

111. Jahanbakhsh, S. P., A. A. Manteghi, S. A. Emami, et al. "Evaluation of the efficacy of Withania somnifera (Ashwagandha) root extract in patients with obsessive-compulsive disorder: A randomized double-blind placebo-controlled trial." *Complementary Therapies in Medicine* 27 (2016): 25–29.

112. Jain, J., V. Narayanan, S. Chaturvedi, S. Pai and S. Sunil. "In vivo evaluation of Withania somnifera–Based Indian traditional formulation (amukkara choornam), against chikungunya virus–induced morbidity and arthralgia." *Journal of Evidence-Based Integrative Medicine* 23, (2018): 1–7. DOI: 10.1177/2156587218757661

113. Jamal, S. A., S. Qureshi, S. N. Ali, M. I. Choudhary and A. U. Rahman. "Bioactivities and structural studies of withanolides from Withania somnifera." *Chemistry of Heterocyclic Compounds* 31, no. 9 (1995): 1047–1059.

114. Jayaprakasam, B. and M. G. Nair. "Cyclooxygenase-2 enzyme inhibitory witha-nolides from Withania somnifera leaves." *Tetrahedron* 59, no. 6 (2003): 841–849.

115. Jayaprakasam, B., G. A. Strasburg and M. G. Nair. "Potent lipid inhibitors from Withania somnifera fruits." *Tetrahedron* 60, no. 13 (2004): 3109–3121.

116. Jayaprakasam, B., K. Padmanabhan and M. G. Nair. "Withanamides in Withania somnifera fruit protect PC-12 cells from beta-amyloid responsible for Alzheimer's disease." *Phytotherapy Research* 24, no. 6 (2010): 859–863.

117. Jirge, S. S., P. A. Tatke and S. Y. Gabhe. "Development and validation of a novel HPTLC method for simultaneous estimation of betasitosterol-D-glucoside and withaferin A." *International Journal of Pharmacy & Pharmaceutical Sciences* 3, no. S2 (2011): 227–230.

118. Joshi, C., N. Gajbhiye, A. Phurailatpam, K. A. Geetha and S. Maiti. "Comparative morphometric, physiological and chemical studies of wild and cultivated plant types of Withania somnifera." *Current Science* 99, no. 3 (2010): 644–650.

119. Joshi, R. A. "Ashwagandha (Withania somnifera) as anticancer herb: An overview." *International Journal of Pharmaceutical Research and Bio-Science* 6, no. 1 (2017): 74–92.

120. Kalaichelvi, K. and A. A. Swaminathan. "Alternate land use through cultivation of medicinal and aromatic plants—A review." *Agricultural Reviews* 30 (2009): 176–183.

121. Kalra, R. and N. Kaushik. "Withania somnifera (Linn.) Dunal: A review of chemical and pharmacological diversity." *Phytochemical Review* 16, no. 5 (2017): 953–987.

122. Kandil, F. E., N. H. El Sayed, A. M. Abou-Douh, M. S. Ishak and T. J. Mabry. "Flavonol glycosides and phenolics from Withania somnifera." *Phytochemistry* 37, no. 4 (1994): 1215–1216.

123. Kapur, L. D. *Handbook of Ayurvedic Medicinal Plants*, London: CRC Press (2001).

124. Kashyap, V. K., A. Dhasmana, M. M. Yallapu, S. C. Chauhan and M. Jaggi. "Withania somnifera as a potential future drug molecule for COVID-19." *Future Drug Discovery* 2, no. 4 (2020): FDD50.

125. Kaul, S. C. and R. Wadhwa Ed. *Science of Ashwagandha: Preventive and Therapeutic Potentials*, Springer Nature, Cham, Switzerland (2017):81–103.

126. Kaul, M. K., A. Kumar, A. Ahuja, B. A. Mir, K. A. Suri and G. N. Qazi. "Production dynamics of withaferin A in Withania somnifera (L.) Dunal complex." *Natural Product Research* 23, no. 14 (2009): 1304–1311.

127. Kaur, S., K. Chauhan and H. Sachdeva. "Protection against experimental visceral leishmaniasis by immunostimulation with herbal drugs derived from Withania somnifera and Asparagus racemosus." *Journal of Medical Microbiology* 63, no. 10 (2014): 1328–3138.

128. Kaur, T., H. Singh, R. Mishra, et al. "Withania somnifera as a potential anxiolytic and immunomodulatory agent in acute sleep deprived female Wistar rats." *Molecular and Cellular Biochemistry* 427, no. 1–2 (2017): 91–101.

129. Kaurav, B. P., M. M. Wanjari, A. Chandekar, N. S. Chauhan and N. Upmanyu. "Influence of Withania somnifera on obsessive compulsive disorder in mice." *Asian Pacific Journal of Tropical Medicine* 5, no. 5 (2012): 380–384.

130. Kaushik, M. K., S. C. Kaul, R. Wadhwa, M. Yanagisawa and Y. Urade. "Triethylene glycol, an active component of Ashwagandha (Withania somnifera) leaves, is responsible for sleep induction." *PLoS One* 12, no. 2 (2017): e0172508.

131. Keche, Y., V. Badar and M. Hardas. "Efficacy and safety of livwin (polyherbal formulation) in patients with acute viral hepatitis: A randomized double-blind placebo-controlled clinical trial." *International Journal of Ayurveda Research* 1, no. 4 (2010): 216–219.

132. Kelgane, S. B., J. Salve, P. Sampara and K. Debnath. "Efficacy and tolerability of Ashwagandha root extract in the elderly for improvement of general well-being and sleep: A prospective, randomized, double-blind, placebo-controlled study." *Cureus* 12, no. 2 (2020): e7083. doi: 10.7759/cureus.7083

133. Khajuria, R. K., K. A. Suri, R. K. Gupta, N. K. Satti, M. Amina, O. P. Suri and G. N. Qazi. "Separation, identification, and quantification of selected withanolides in plant extracts of Withania somnifera by HPLC-UV (DAD)-positive ion electrospray ionisation-mass spectrometry." *Journal of Separation Science* 27, no. 7–8 (2004): 541–546.

134. Khan, M. A., R. A. Ahmed, N. Chandra, V. K. Arora and A. Ali. "In vivo, extract from Withania somnifera root ameliorates arthritis via regulation of key immune mediators of inflammation in experimental model of arthritis." *Anti-inflammatory & Anti-allergy Agents in Medicinal Chemistry* 18, no. 1 (2019): 55–70.

135. Khanchandani, N., P. Shah, T. Kalwani, A. Ardeshna and D. Dharajiya. "Antibacterial and antifungal activity of Ashwagandha (Withania somnifera l.): A review." *Journal of Drug Delivery and Therapeutics* 9, no. 5-s (2019): 154–161.

136. Khare, C. "Withania Ashwagandha Kaul (cultivated var.)." In C. Khare (ed.) *Indian Medicinal Plants*, New York, NY: Springer (2007).

137. Khedgikar, V., N. Ahmad and P. Kushwaha, et al. "Preventive effects of withaferin A isolated from the leaves of an Indian medicinal plant Withania somnifera (L.): Comparisons with 17-β-estradiol and alendronate." *Nutrition* 31, no. 1 (2015): 205–213.

138. Kim, S.-K., K. B. Singh, E.-R. Hahm, B. L. Lokeshwar and S. V. Singh. "Withania somnifera root extract inhibits fatty acid synthesis in prostate cancer cells." *Journal of Traditional and Complementary Medicine* 10 (2020): 188–197.

139. Kim, S., J. S. Yu, J. Y. Lee, S. U. Choi, J. Lee and K. H. Kim. "Cytotoxic withanolides from the roots of Indian ginseng (Withania somnifera)." *Journal of Natural Products* 82, no. 4 (2019): 765–773.

140. Kirtikar, K. R. and B. D. Basu. *Indian Medicinal Plants*, Vol. II, Allahabad: Lalit Mohan Basu Publication (1935): 1774–1776.

141. Konar, A., N. Shah, R. Singh, et al. "Protective role of Ashwagandha leaf extract and its component withanone on scopolamine-induced changes in the brain and brain-derived cells." *PLoS One* 6, no. 11 (2011): e27265.

142. Koval, L., N. Zemskaya, A. Aliper, A. Zhavoronkov and A. Moskalev. "Evaluation of the geroprotective effects of withaferin A in drosophila melanogaster." *Aging (Albany NY)* 13, no. 2 (2021): 1817–1841.

143. Krutika, J., S. Tavhare, K. Panara, P. Kumar and N. Karra. "Studies of Ashwagandha (Withania somnifera Dunal." *International Journal of Pharmaceutical & Biological Archives* 7, no. 1 (2016): 1–11.

144. Kuboyama, T., C. Tohda and K. Komatsu. "Withanoside IV and its active metabolite, sominone, attenuate abeta (25-35)-induced neurodegeneration." *European Journal of Neuroscience* 23, no. 6 (2006): 1417–1426.

145. Kuchewar, V. V., M. A. Borkar and M. A. Nisargandha. "Evaluation of anti-oxidant potential of rasayana drugs in healthy human volunteers." *Ayu* 35, no. 1 (2014): 46–49.

146. Kulkarni, R. R., P. S. Patki and V. P. Jog. "Treatment of osteoarthritis with a herbomineral formulation: A double-blind, placebo-controlled, cross-over study." *Journal of Ethnopharmacology* 33, no. 1–2 (1991): 91–95.

147. Kulkarni, S. N. and A. Dhir. "Withania somnifera: An Indian ginseng." *Progress in Neuro-Psychopharmacology & Biological Psychiatry* 32, no. 5 (2008): 1093–1105.

148. Kumar, S., R. Singh, N. Gajbhiye and T. Dhanani. "Extraction optimization for phenolic- and withanolide-rich fractions from Withania somnifera roots: Identification and quantification of withaferin a, 12-deoxywithastromonolide, and withanolide a in plant materials and marketed formulations using a reversed-phase HPLC-photodiode array detection method." *Journal of AOAC International* 10, no. 6 (2018): 1773–1780.

149. Kumar, A. and H. Kalonia. "Effect of Withania somnifera on sleep-wake cycle in sleep-disturbed rats: Possible GABAergic mechanism." *Indian Journal of Pharmaceutical Sciences* 70, no. 6 (2008): 806–810.

150. Kumar, A., M. Kaul, M. Bhan, P. Khanna and K. Suri. "Morphological and chemical variation in 25 collections of the Indian medicinal plant, Withania somnifera (L.) Dunal (Solanaceae)." *Genetic Resources and Crop Evolution* 54, (2007): 655–660.

151. Kumar, G., A. Srivastava, S. K. Sharma, T. D. Rao and Y. K. Gupta. "Efficacy and safety evaluation of Ayurvedic treatment (Ashwagandha powder & Sidh Makardhwaj) in rheumatoid arthritis patients: A pilot prospective study." *Journal of Medical Research* 141, no. 1 (2015b): 100–106.

152. Kumar, P. and A. Kumar. "Possible neuroprotective effect of Withania somnifera root extract against 3-nitropropionic acid-induced behavioral, biochemical, and mitochondrial dysfunction in an animal model of Huntington's disease." *Journal of Medicinal Food* 12, no. 3 (2009): 591–600.

153. Kumar, R., K. Gupta, K. Saharia, D. Pradhan and J. R. Subramaniam. "Withania somnifera root extract extends lifespan of caenorhabditis elegans." *Annals of Neurosciences* 20, no. 1 (2013): 13–16.

154. Kumar, S., G. J. Dobos and T. Rampp. "The significance of Ayurvedic medicinal plants." *Journal of Evidence-based Complementary & Alternative Medicine* 22, no. 3 (2017): 494–501.

155. Kumar, V., A. Dey, M. B. Hadimani, T. Marcović and M. Emerald. "Chemistry and pharmacology of Withania somnifera: An update." *TANG (Humanitas Medicine)* 5, no. 1 (2015a): 1–13.

156. Kumar, V., J. K. Dhanjal, P. Bhargava., et al. "Withanone and withaferin-A are predicted to interact with transmembrane protease serine 2 (TMPRSS2) and block entry of SARS-CoV-2 into cells." *Journal of Biomolecular Structure & Dynamics* 2020 (2020): 1–13. doi.org/10.1080/07391102.2020.1775704

157. Kuttan, G. "Use of Withania somnifera Dunal as an adjuvant during radiation therapy." *Indian Journal of Experimental Biology* 34, no. 9 (1996): 854–856.

158. Lal, P., L. N. Misra, R. S. Sangwan and R. Tuli. "New withanolides from fresh berries of Withania somnifera." *Zeitschrift für Naturforschung B* 61, no. 9 (2006): 1143–1147.

159. Langade, D., S. Kanchi and J. Salve, et al. "Efficacy and safety of Ashwagandha (Withania somnifera) root extract in insomnia and anxiety: A double-blind, randomized, placebo-controlled study." *Cureus* 11, no. 9 (2019): e5797.

160. Lavie, D., E. Glotter and Y. Shvo. "Constituents of Withania somnifera dun. Part IV. The structure of withaferin A." *Journal of the Chemical Society* (1965): 7517–7531.

161. Lee, I.-C. and B. Y. Choi. "Withaferin-A—A natural anticancer agent with pleitropic mechanisms of action." *International Journal of Molecular Sciences* 17, no. 3 (2016): 290.

162. Logie, E. and W. V. Berghe. "Tackling chronic inflammation with withanolide phytochemicals—A withaferin A perspective" *Antioxidants* 9 (2020): 1107. doi: 10.3390/antiox9111107

163. Lopresti, A. L., P. D. Drummond and S. J. Smith. "A randomized, double-blind, placebo-controlled, crossover study examining the hormonal and vitality effects of Ashwagandha (Withania somnifera) in aging, overweight males." *American Journal of Men's Health* 13, no. 2 (2019a): 1–15. https://doi.org/10.1177/1557988319835985

164. Lopresti, A. L., S. J. Smith, H. Malvi and R. Kodgule. "An investigation into the stress-relieving and pharmacological actions of an Ashwagandha (Withania somnifera) extract. A randomized, double-blind, placebo-controlled study." *Medicine* 98, no. 37 (2019b): e17186. dx.doi.org/10.1097/MD.0000000000017186

165. Machiah, D. K., K. S. Girish and T. V. Gowda. "A glycoprotein from a folk medicinal plant, Withania somnifera, inhibits hyaluronidase activity of snake venoms." *Comparative Biochemistry and Physiology, Toxicology and Pharmacology* 143, no. 2 (2006): 158–161.

166. Mahrous, R. S. R., D. A. Ghareeb, H. M. Fathy, R. M. Abu EL-Khair and A. A. Omar. "The protective effect of Egyptian Withania somnifera against Alzheimer's." *Medicinal and Aromatic Plants* 6, no. 2 (2017): 1000285.

167. Mahrous, R. S. R., H. M. Fathy, R. M. Abu EL-Khair and A. A. Omar. "Chemical constituents of Egyptian Withania somnifera leaves and fruits and their anticholinesterase activity." *Journal of the Mexican Chemical Society* 63, no. 4 (2019): 208–217.

168. Majumdar, D. N. "Withania somnifera Dunal, part II, alkaloidal constituents and their chemical characterization." *Indian Journal of Pharmacology* 17, (1955): 158–161.

169. Manohar, P. R. "Clinical evidence in the tradition of Ayurveda." In S. Rastogi (ed.) *Evidence-Based Practice in Complementary and Alternative Medicine*, Heidelberg: Springer (2012): 67–78.

170. Mansour, H. H. and H. F. Hafez. "Protective effect of Withania somnifera against radiation-induced hepatotoxicity in rats." *Ecotoxicology Environmental Safety* 80 (2012): 14–19.

171. Marell, P. and J. Brar. "SU66 pilot study on the effects of Withania somnifera on electrophysiological measures of sensory and cognitive processing in schizophrenia." *Schizophrenia Bulletin* 43, no. S1 (2017): S185.

172. Matsuda, H., T. Murakami, A. Kishi and M. Yoshikawa. "Structures of withanosides I, II, III, IV, V, VI, and VII, new withanolide glycosides, from the roots of Indian Withania somnifera DUNAL and inhibitory activity for tachyphylaxis to clonidine in isolated Guinea-pig ileum." *Bioorganic and Medicinal Chemistry* 9, no. 6 (2001): 1499–1507.

173. Mehta, V., H. Chander and A. Munshi. "Mechanisms of anti-tumor activity of Withania somnifera (Ashwagandha)". *Nutrition and Cancer* 73, no. 6 (2020): 1–13. doi:10.1080/01635581.2020.1778746

174. Minhas, U., R. Minz, P. Das and A. Bhatnagar. "Therapeutic effect of Withania somnifera on pristane-induced model of SLE." *Inflammopharmacology* 20, no. 4 (2012): 195–205.

175. Mir, B. A., J. Khazir, N. A. Mir, T.-U Hasan and S. Koul. "Botanical, chemical and pharmacological review of Withania somnifera (Indian ginseng): An Ayurvedic medicinal plant." *Indian Journal of Drugs and Diseases* 1, no. 6 (2012): 147–160.

176. Mirjalili, M. H., A. Navarro, L. Hernandez, O. Jauregui and M. Bonfill. "LC–MS/MS method for the quantification of withaferin-a in plant extracts of Withania spp." *Acta Chromatographica* 25, no. 4 (2013): 745–754.

177. Mirjalili, M. H., E. Moyano, M. Bonfill, R. M. Cusido and J. Palazon. "Steroidal lactones from Withania somnifera, an ancient plant for novel medicine." *Molecules* 14 (2009a): 2373–2393.

178. Mirjalili, M. H., S. M. Fakhr-Tabatabaei, H. Alizadeh, A. Ghassempour and F. Mirzajani. "Genetic and withaferin A analysis of Iranian natural populations of Withania somnifera and W. Coagulans by RAPD and HPTLC." *Natural Product Communications* 4, no. 3 (2009b): 337–346.

179. Mishra, B. *Ashwagandha – Bhavprakash Nigantu (Indian Materia Medica)*, Varanasi: Chaukhambha Bharti Academy (2004): 393–394.

180. Mishra, L. C., B. B. Singh and S. Dagenais. "Scientific basis for the therapeutic use of Withania somnifera (Ashwagandha): A review." *Alternative Medicine Review* 5, no. 4 (2000): 334–346.

181. Misico, R. I., V. E. Nicotra, J. C. Oberti, G. Barboza, R. R. Gil and G. Burton "Withanolides and related steroids." In A. Kinghorn, H. Falk and J. Kobayashi (eds.) *Progress in the Chemistry of Organic Natural Products*, Vol. 94, Vienna: Springer (2011).

182. Misra, L. N., P. Lal, R. S. Sangwan, N. S. Sangwan, G. C. Uniyal and R. Tuli. "Unusually sulfated and oxygenated steroids from Withania somnifera." *Phytochemistry* 66, no. 23 (2005): 2702–2707.

183. Misra, L. N., P. Mishra, A. Pandey, R. Sangwan, N. Sangwan and R. Tuli. "Withanolides from Withania somnifera roots." *Phytochemistry* 69, no. 4 (2008): 1000–1004.

184. Misra, L., P. Mishra, A. Pandey, R. S. Sangwan and N. S. Sangwan. "1, 4-dioxane and ergosterol derivatives from Withania somnifera roots." *Journal of Asian Natural Products Research* 14, no. 1 (2012): 39–45.

185. Mohan, R., H. J. Hammers, P. Bargagna-Mohan, X. H. Zhan, C. J. Herbstritt and A. Ruiz. "Withaferin A is a potent inhibitor of angiogenesis." *Angiogenesis* 7, (2004): 115–122.

186. Mohanty, I. R., D. S. Arya and S. K. Gupta. "Withania somnifera provides cardioprotection and attenuates ischemia-reperfusion induced apoptosis." *Clinical Nutrition* 27, no. 4 (2008): 635–642.

187. Mukherjee, P. K., S. Banerjee, S. Biswas, B. Das, A. Kar and K. C. Katiyar. "Withania somnifera (L.) dunal—Modern perspectives of an ancient rasayana from Ayurveda". *Journal of Ethnopharmacology* 264 (2021): 113157.

188. Mundkinajeddu, D., L. P. Swant, and R. Koshy, et al. "Development and validation of high performance liquid chromatography method for simultaneous estimation of flavonoid glycosides in Withania somnifera aerial parts." *International
Scholarly Research Notices Analytical Chemistry* 2014, no. 6 (2014): Article ID
351547. doi.org/10.1155/2014/351547

189. Murthy, M. N. K., S. Gundagani, C. Nutalapati and U. Pingali. "Evaluation of
analgesic activity of standardised aqueous extract of Withania somnifera in
healthy human volunteers using mechanical pain model." *Journal of Clinical
and Diagnostic Research* 13, no. 1 (2019): FC01–FC04.

190. Murthy, M. R. V., P. K. Ranjekar, C. Ramassamy and M. Deshpande. "Scientific
basis for the use of Indian Ayurvedic medicinal plants in the treatment of neurodegenerative disorders: Ashwagandha." *Central Nervous System Agents in
Medicinal Chemistry* 10, no. 3 (2010): 238–246.

191. Musharraf, S. G., A. Ali, R. A. Ali, S. Yousuf, A. U. Rahman and M. I.
Choudhary. "Analysis and development of structure-fragmentation relationships
in withanolides using an electrospray ionization quadrupole time-of-flight tandem mass spectrometry hybrid instrument." *Rapid Communications in Mass
Spectrometry* 25, no. 1 (2011): 104–114.

192. Musharraf, S. G., A. Ali and M. I. Choudhary. "Atta-ur-Rahman. Probing of
metabolites in finely powdered plant material by direct laser desorption ionization mass spectrometry." *Journal of the American Society for Mass Spectrometry*
25, no. 4 (2014): 530–537.

193. Mwitari, P. G., P. A. Ayeka, J. Ondicho, E. N. Matu and C. C. Bii. "Antimicrobial
activity and probable mechanisms of action of medicinal plants of Kenya:
Withania somnifera, Warbugia ugandensis, Prunus africana and Plectrunthus
barbatus." *PLoS One* 8, no. 6 (2013): e65619.

194. Nagappan, A., N. Karunanithi, S. Sentrayaperumal, et al. "Comparative root protein profiles of Korean ginseng (Panax ginseng) and Indian ginseng (Withania
somnifera)." *The American Journal of Chinese Medicine* 40, no. 1 (2012): 203–218.

195. Nair, A. R. and N. Praveen. "Biochemical and phytochemical variations during
the growth phase of Withania somnifera (L.) Dunal." *Journal of Pharmacognosy
and Phytochemistry* 8, no. 3 (2019): 1930–1937.

196. Namdeo, A. G., A. Sharma, K. N. Yadav, et al. "Metabolic characterization of
Withania somnifera from different regions of India using NMR spectroscopy."
Planta Medica 77 (2011): 1058–1964.

197. Narinderpal, K., N. Junaid and B. Raman. "A review on pharmacological profile of Withania somnifera (Ashwagandha)." *Research and reviews." Journal of
Botanical Sciences* 2, no. 4 (2013): 6–14.

198. Ng, Q. F., W. Loke and N. X. Foo, et al. "A systematic review of the clinical
use of Withania somnifera (Ashwagandha) to ameliorate cognitive dysfunction."
Phytotherapy Research 34, no. 3 (2020): 583–590.

199. Nile, A. H. and S. W. Park. "HPTLC densitometry method for simultaneous
determination of flavonoids in selected medicinal plants." *Frontiers in Life
Science* 8, no. 1 (2015): 97–103.

200. Nile, S. H., A. Nile, E. Gansukh, V. Baskar and G. Kai. "Subcritical water extraction of withanosides and withanolides from Ashwagandha (Withania somnifera
L) and their biological activities" *Food and Chemical Toxicology* 132 (2019):
110659. doi: 10.1016/j.fct.2019.110659

201. Palliyaguru, D. L., S. V. Singh and T. W. Kensler. "Withania somnifera: From prevention to treatment of cancer." *Molecular Nutrition & Food Research* 60, no. 6 (2016): 1342–1353.

202. Patel, B. H., J. B. Patel and R. K. Patel. "Novel validated HPTLC method for estimation of withaferin A in polyherbal formulations." *Analytical Methods* 6, no. 9 (2014): 3009–3012.

203. Patel, K., R. B. Singh and D. K. Patel. "Pharmacological and analytical aspects of withaferin A: A concise report of current scientific literature." *Asian Pacific Journal of Reproduction* 2, no. 3 (2013): 238–243.

204. Patil, D., M. Gautam, S. Mishra, et al. "Determination of withaferin A and withanolide A in mice plasma using high-performance liquid chromatography-tandem mass spectrometry: Application to pharmacokinetics after oral administration of Withania somnifera aqueous extract." *Journal of Pharmaceutical and Biomedical Analysis* 80 (2013): 203–212.

205. Patwardhan, B., G. T. Panse and P. H. Kulkarni. "Ashwagandha (Withania somnifera): A review." *Journal of National Integrated Medical Association* 30, no. 6 (1988): 7–11.

206. Pawar, P., S. Gilda, S. Sharma, et al. "Rectal gel application of Withania somnifera root extract expounds anti-inflammatory and muco-restorative activity in TNBS-induced inflammatory bowel disease." *BMC Complementary and Alternative Medicine* 11 (2011): 34.

207. Penman, K., T. Briski, K. M. Bone, et al. "Withania somnifera HPLC-PDA method validation." *Planta Medica* 73 (2007): P_251 DOI: 10.1055/s-2007-987032

208. Pérez-Gómez, P. J., S. Villafaina, J. C. Adsuar, E. Merellano-Navarro and D. Collado-Mateo. "Effects of Ashwagandha (Withania somnifera) on VO_{2max}: A systematic review and meta-analysis." *Nutrients* 12, no. 4 (2020): 1119. doi:10.3390/nu12041119

209. Petrovska, B. B. "Historical review of medicinal plants' usage." *Pharmacognosy Reviews* 6, no. 11 (2012): 1–5.

210. Philips, C. A., R. Ahamed, S. Rajesh, T. George, M. Mohanan and P. Augustine. "Comprehensive review of hepatotoxicity associated with traditional Indian Ayurvedic herbs." *World Journal of Hepatology* 12, no. 9 (2020): 574–595.

211. Pingali, U., R. Pilli and N. Fatima. "Effect of standardized aqueous extract of Withania somnifera on tests of cognitive and psychomotor performance in healthy human participants." *Pharmacognosy Research* 6, no. 1 (2014): 12–18.

212. Powell, D., T. Inoue, G. Bahtiyar, G. Fenteany and A. Sacerdote. "Treatment of nonclassic 11-hydroxylase deficiency with Ashwagandha root." *Case Reports in Endocrinology* 2017 (2017): 1869560.

213. Prakash, J., S. K. Gupta and A. K. Dinda. "Withania somnifera root extract prevents DMBA-induced squamous cell carcinoma of skin in Swiss albino mice." *Nutrition and Cancer* 42, no. 1 (2002): 91–97.

214. Prakash, J., S. K. Yadav, S. Chouhan and S. P. Singh. "Neuroprotective role of Withania somnifera root extract in maneb-paraquat induced mouse model of parkinsonism." *Neurochemical Research* 38, no. 5 (2013): 972–980.

215. Pratibha, C., M. Bora and A. Parihar. "Therapeutic properties and significance of different parts of Ashwagandha-A medicinal plant." *International Journal of Pure & Applied Bioscience* 1, no. 6 (2013): 94–101.

216. Pratte, M. A., K. B. Nanavati, V. Young and C. P. Morley. "An alternative treatment for anxiety: A systematic review of human trial results reported for the Ayurvedic herb Ashwagandha (Withania somnifera)." *Journal of Alternative and Complementary Medicine* 20, no. 12 (2014): 901–908.

217. Purdie, R. W., D. E. Symon and L. Haegi. "Solanaceae." *Flora of Australia* 29 (1982): 184–186.

218. Puri, H. S. *Simple Ayurvedic Remedies*, New Delhi: UBS Publishers Distributors (2002).

219. Quattrocchi, U. *CRC World Dictionary of Medicinal and Poisonous Plants: Common Names, Scientific Names, Eponyms, Synonyms and Etymology.* Boca Raton, Florida: CRC Press, Taylor and Francis Group (2012).

220. Raguraman, V. and J. Subramaniam. "Withania somnifera root extract enhances telomerase activity in the human HeLa cell line." *Advances in Bioscience and Biotechnology* 7 (2016): 199–204.

221. Rahmati, B., M. H. G. Moghaddam, M. Khalili, E. Enayati, M. Maleki and S. Rezaeei. "Effect of Withania somnifera (L.) Dunal on sex hormone and gonadotropin levels in addicted male rats." *International Journal of Fertility and Sterility* 10, no. 2 (2016): 239–244. doi:10.22074/ijfs.2016.4915

222. Rai, M., P. S. Jogee, G. Agarkar and C. A. dos Santos. "Anticancer activities of Withania somnifera: Current research, formulations, and future perspectives." *Pharmaceutical Biology* 54, no. 2 (2016): 189–197.

223. Raju, S. K., P. L. Basavanna, H. N. Nagesh and A. D. Shanbhag. "A study on the anticonvulsant activity of Withania somnifera (Dunal) in albino rats." *National Journal of Physiology, Pharmacy and Pharmacology* 7, no. 1 (2017): 17–21.

224. Ramakanth, G. S., C. Uday Kumar, P. V. Kishan, et al. "A randomized, double blind placebo controlled study of efficacy and tolerability of Withania somnifera extracts in knee joint pain." *Journal of Ayurveda and Integrated Medicine* 7, no. 3 (2016): 151–157.

225. Rasool, M. and P. Varalakshmi. "Immunomodulatory role of Withania somnifera root powder on experimental induced inflammation: An in vivo and in vitro study." *Vascular Pharmacology* 44, no. 6 (2006): 406–410.

226. Ray, A. B. and M. Gupta "Withasteroids, a growing group of naturally occurring steroidal lactones". In W. Herz, G. W. Kirby, R. E. Moore, W. Steglich and C. Tamm (eds.) *Progress in the Chemistry of Organic Natural Products.* Vol. 63, Vienna: Springer (1994).

227. Rayees, S. and F. Malik. "Withania somnifera: From traditional use to vidence based medicinal prominence." In S. Kaul R. Wadhwa (eds.) *Science of Ashwagandha: Preventive and Therapeutic Potentials*, Cham: Springer International Publishing AG (2017).

228. Rege, N. N., U. M. Thatte and S. A. Dahanukar. "Adaptogenic properties of six rasayana herbs used in Ayurvedic medicine." *Phytotherapy Research* 13, no. 4 (1999): 275–291.

229. Rohma, G., B. Admasu, T. H. Gebrekidan, H. Aleme and G. Gebru. "Antibacterial activities of five medicinal plants in Ethiopia against some human and animal pathogens." *Evidence-Based Complementary and Alternative Medicine* 2018 (2018): Article ID 2950758.

230. Saggam, A., G. Tillu, S. Dixit, et al. "Withania somnifera (L.) Dunal: A potential therapeutic adjuvant in cancer." *Journal of Ethnopharmacology* 255 (2020): 112759. doi: 10.1016/j.jep.2020.112759

231. Saleem, S., G. Muhammad, M. A. Hussain, M. Altaf and S. N. A. Bukhari "Withania somnifera L.: Insights into the phytochemical profile, therapeutic potential, clinical trials, and future prospective." *Iran Journal of Basic Medical Science* 23 (2020):1501–1526.

232. Salve, J., S. Pate, K. Debnath, et al. "Adaptogenic and anxiolytic effects of Ashwagandha root extract in healthy adults: A double-blind, randomized, placebo-controlled clinical study." *Cureus* 11, no. 12 (2019): e6466. doi: 10.7759/cureus.6466

233. Samadi, A. K. "Ashwagandha: ancient medicine for modern times." *Journal of Ancient Diseases Preventive Remedies* 1, no. 3 (2013): 1000e108.

234. Sandhu, J. S., B. Shah, S. Shenoy, S. Chauhan, G. S. Lavekar and M. M. Padhi. "Effects of Withania somnifera (Ashwagandha) and Terminalia arjuna (Arjuna) on physical performance and cardiorespiratory endurance in healthy young adults." *International Journal of Ayurveda Research* 1, no. 3 (2010): 144–149.

235. Sangwan, N. S., S. Tripathi, Y. Srivastava, B. Mishra and N. Pandey. "Phytochemical genomics of Ashwagandha." In S. C. Kaul and R. Wadhwa (eds.) *Science of Ashwagandha: Preventive and Therapeutic Potentials*, Cham, Switzerland: Springer Nature (2017): 3–36.

236. Sangwan, R. S., N. D. Chaurasia, L. N. Misra, et al. "Phytochemical variability in commercial herbal products and preparations of Withania somnifera (Ashwagandha)." *Current Science* 86, no. 3 (2004): 461–465.

237. Sangwan, R. S., N. D. Chaurasiya, P. Lal, L. Misra, R. Tuli and N. S. Sangwan. "Withanolide A is inherently de novo biosynthesized in roots of the medicinal plant Ashwagandha (Withania somnifera)." *Physiologia Plantarum* 133, no. 2 (2008): 278–287.

238. Saritha, K. V. and C. V. Naidu. "In vitro flowering of Withania somnifera Dunal. An important antitumor medicinal plant." *Plant Science* 172, no. 4 (2007): 847–851.

239. Sayantan, G. and L. Sujata. "Withanolide D of Ashwagandha improves apoptosis in the bone marrow of leukemic murine model." *Journal of Biomedical Research and Environmental Science* 2, no. 6 (2021): 431–438.

240. Schröter, H.-B., D. Neumann, A. R. Katritzky and F. J. Swinbourne. "Withasomnine. A pyrazole alkaloid from Withania somnifera dun." *Tetrahedron* 22, no. 8 (1966): 2895–2897.

241. Schwarting, A. E., J. M. Bobbitt, A. Rother, et al. "The alkaloids of Withania somnifera.".*Lloydia* 26 (1963): 258–273.

242. Sehgal, N., A. Gupta, R. K. Valli, et al. "Withania somnifera reverses Alzheimer's disease pathology by enhancing low-density lipoprotein receptor-related protein in liver." *Proceedings of National Academy of Sciences USA* 109, no. 9 (2012): 3510–3515.

243. Sengupta, P., A. Agarwal, M. Pogrebetskaya, S. Roychoudhury, D. Durairajanayagam and R. Henkel. "Role of Withania somnifera (Ashwagandha) in the management of male infertility." *Reproductive Biomedicine Online* 36 (2018): 311–326.

244. Senthil, K., N. Karunanithi, G. S. Kim, et al. "Proteome analysis of in vitro and in vivo root tissue of Withania somnifera." *African Journal of Biotechnology* 10, no. 74 (2011): 16875–16883.

245. Senthil, K., P. Thirugnanasambantham, T. J. Oh, S. H. Kim and H. K. Choi. "Free radical scavenging activity and comparative metabolic profiling of in vitro cultured and field grown Withania somnifera roots. *PLoS ONE* 10, no. 4 (2015): e0123360.

246. Shah, D. R., S. J. Palaskar, R. B. Pawar and R. R. Punse. "Withania somnifera: A new approach to cancer." *Annals of Applied Bio-Sciences* 5, no. 1 (2018): R1–R8.

247. Shah, N., R. Singh and U. Sarangi. "Combinations of Ashwagandha leaf extracts protect brain-derived cells against oxidative stress and induce differentiation." *PLoS One* 10, no. 3 (2015): e0120554.

248. Shahraki, M. R., Z. Samadi Noshahr, H. Ahmadvand and A. Nakhaie. "Antinociceptive and anti-inflammatory effects of Withania somnifera root in fructose fed male rats." *Journal of Basic and Clinical Physiology and Pharmacology* 27, no. 4 (2016): 387–391.

249. Shalini, R., J. K. Eapen and M. S. Deepa. "Macroscopic evaluation of genuine and market samples of Ashwagandha (Withania somnifera (Linn.) Dunal) in Kerala." *Journal of Pharmacognosy and Phytochemistry* 6, no. 6 (2017): 2283–2288.

250. Sharma, A. K., I. Basu and S. Singh. "Efficacy and safety of Ashwagandha root extract in subclinical hypothyroid patients: A double-blind, randomized placebo-controlled trial." *Journal of Alternative and Complementary Medicine* 24, no. 3 (2018): 243–248.

251. Sharma, R. A., M. Goswami and A. Yadav. "GC-MS screening of alkaloids of Withania somnifera L. in vivo and in vitro." *Indian Journal of Applied Research* 3, no. 8 (2013): 63–66.

252. Sharma, V. "HPLC-PDA method for quantification of withaferin-A and withanolide-A in diploid (n=12) and tetraploid (n=24) cytotypes of 'Indian Ginseng' Withania somnifera (L.) Dunal from North India." *International Journal of Indigenous Medicinal Plants* 46, no. 2 (2013): 1245–1250.

253. Sharma, V., A. P. Gupta, P. Bhandari, R. C. Gupta and B. Singh. "A validated and densitometric HPTLC method for the quantification of withaferin-A and withanolide-A in different plant parts of two morphotypes of Withania somnifera." *Chromatographia* 66 (2007): 801–804.

254. Shenoy, S., U. Chaskar, J. S. Sandhu and M. M. Paadhi. "Effects of eight-week supplementation of Ashwagandha on cardiorespiratory endurance in elite Indian cyclists." *Journal of Ayurveda and Integrated Medicine* 3, no. 4 (2012): 209–214.

255. Shrivastava, A. K. and P. K. Sahu. "Economics of yield and production of alkaloid of Withania somnifera (L.) Dunal." *American Journal of Plant Sciences* 4 (2013): 2023–2030.

256. Siddiqui, S., N. Ahmed, M. Goswami, A. Chakrabarty and G. Chowdhury. "DNA damage by withanone as a potential cause of liver toxicity observed for herbal products of Withania somnifera (Ashwagandha)." *Current Research in Toxicology* 2 (2021): 72–81.

257. Sidhu, O. P., S. Annarao, S. Chatterjee, R. Tuli, R. Roy and C. L. Khetrapal. "Metabolic alterations of Withania somnifera (L.) Dunal fruits at different developmental stages by NMR spectroscopy." *Phytochemical Analysis* 22, no. 6 (2011): 492–502.

258. Silva, R., N. P. Lopes and D. B. Silva. "Application of MALDI mass spectrometry in natural products analysis." *Planta Medica* 82 (2016): 671–689.

259. Singh, M., P. Shah, H. Punetha and S. Agrawal. "Varietal comparison of withanolide contents in different tissues of Withania somnifera (L.) Dunal (Ashwagandha)." *International Journal of Life Sciences and Scientific Research* 4, no. 3 (2018a): 1752–1758.

260. Singh, V., B. Singh, R. Joshi, P. Jaju and P. K. Pati. "Changes in the leaf proteome profile of Withania somnifera (L.) Dunal in response to alternaria alternata infection." *PLoS One* 12, no. 6 (2017): e0178924.

261. Singh, A., V. Bajpai, S. Kumar, K. R. Sharma and B. Kumar. "Profiling of gallic and ellagic acid derivatives in different plant parts of Terminalia arjuna by HPLC-ESI-QTOF-MS/MS." *Natural Product Communications* 11, no. 2 (2016): 239–244.

262. Singh, A., S. Duggal, H. Singh, J. Singh and S. Katekhaye. "Withanolides: Phytoconstituents with significant pharmacological activities." *International Journal of Green Pharmacy* 4, no. 4 (2010a): 229–237.

263. Singh, G., P. K. Sharma, R. Dudhe and S. Singh. "Biological activities of Withania somnifera." *Annals of Biological Research* 1, no. 3 (2010b): 56–63.

264. Singh, N., M. Bhalla, P. Jager and M. Gilca. "An overview on Ashwagandha: A rasayana (rejuvenator) of Ayurveda." *African Journal of Traditional, Complementary and Alternative Medicine* 8, no. 5S (2011a): 208–213.

265. Singh, N., P. Verma, B. R. Pandey and M. Gilca. "Role of Withania somnifera in prevention and treatment of cancer: An overview." *International Journal of Pharmaceutical Sciences and Drug Research* 3, no. 4 (2011b): 274–279.

266. Singh, N., S. N. Rai, D. Singh and S. P. Singh. "Withania somnifera shows ability to counter Parkinson's disease: An update." *SOJ Neurology* 2, no. 2 (2015b): 1–4.

267. Singh, P., R. Guleri, V. Singh, et al. Biotechnological interventions in Withania somnifera (L.) Dunal, *Biotechnology and Genetic Engineering Reviews*, 31, no. 1–2 (2015a): 1–20. doi: 10.1080/02648725.2015.1020467

268. Singh, S. K. and K. Rajoria. "Ayurvedic management of chronic constipation in Hirschsprung disease—A case study." *Journal of Ayurveda and Integrated Medicine* 9, no. 2 (2018): 131–135.

269. Singh, S. and S. Kumar. *Withania somnifera: The Indian Ginseng, Ashwagandha*, Lucknow: Central Institute of Medical and Aromatic Plants (1998).

270. Singh, V. K., D. Mundkinajeddu, A. Agarwal, J. Nguyen, S. Sudberg, S. Gafner and M. Blumenthal. "Adulteration of Ashwagandha (Withania somnifera) Roots and Extracts." *Botanical Adulterants Prevention Bulletin*, Austin, TX: ABC-AHP-NCNPR Botanical Adulterants Prevention Program; 2018b. http://www.herbalgram.org/media/13136/bap-babs-ashwa-cc-012019-final.pdf

271. Singh, V., B. Singh, A. Sharma, et al. "Leaf spot disease adversely affects human health-promoting constituents and withanolide biosynthesis in Withania somnifera (L.) Dunal." *Journal of Applied Microbiology* 122, no. 1 (2016): 153–165.

272. Sinha, S., G. Nosál'ová, S. S. Bandyopadhyay, D. Flešková and B. Ray. "In vivo anti-tussive activity and structural features of a polysaccharide fraction from water extracted Withania somnifera." *Ethnopharmacology* 134, no. 2 (2011): 510–513.

273. Siriwardane, A. S., R. M. Dharmadasa and K. Samarasinghe. "Distribution of withaferin A, an anticancer potential agent, in different parts of two varieties of Withania somnifera (L.) Dunal grown in Sri Lanka." *Pakistan Journal of Biological Sciences* 16, no. 3 (2013): 141–144.

274. Sivasankarapillai, V. S., R. M. K. Nair, A. Rahdar, et al. "Overview of the anticancer activity of withaferin A, an active constituent of the Indian ginseng Withania somnifera" *Environmental Science and Pollution Research* 27 (2020): 26025–26035.

275. Sonar, V. P., F. Cottiglia, S. Ruiu, et al. "Withanolides and alkaloids from Withania somnifera roots with binding affinity to opioid, cannabinoids and GABAergic receptors." *Planta Medica* 81 (2015): PW_122.

276. Sood, A., A. Kumar, D. K. Dhawan and R. Sandhir. "Propensity of Withania somnifera to attenuate behavioural, biochemical, and histological alterations in experimental model of stroke." *Cellular and Molecular Neurobiology* 36, no. 7 (2016): 1123–1138.

277. Srivastava, P., N. Tiwari, A. K. Yadav, et al. "Simultaneous quantification of withanolides in Withania somnifera by a validated high-performance thin-layer chromatographic method." *Journal of AOAC International* 91, no. 5 (2008): 1154–1161.

278. Srivastava, A., A. K. Gupta, K. Shanker, M. M. Gupta, R. Mishra and R. K. Lal. "Genetic variability, associations, and path analysis of chemical and morphological traits in Indian ginseng [Withania somnifera (L.) Dunal] for selection of higher yielding genotypes." *Journal of Ginseng Research* 42, no. 2 (2018): 158–164.

279. Srivastava, N. and V. Saxena. "A review on scope of immuno-modulatory drugs in Ayurveda for prevention and treatment of Covid-19." *Plant Science Today* 7, no. 3 (2020): 417–423. https://doi.org/10.14719/pst.2020.7.3.831

280. Straughn, A. R. and S. S. Kakar. "Withaferin A: A potential therapeutic agent against COVID-19 infection " *Journal of Ovarian Research* 13 (2020): 79. doi.org/10.1186/s13048-020-00684-x

281. Subbaraju, G. V., M. Vanisree, C. V. Rao, et al. "Ashwagandhanolide, a bioactive dimeric thiowithanolide isolated from the roots of Withania somnifera." *Journal of Natural Products* 69, no. 12 (2006): 1790–1792.

282. Sumantran, V. N., A. Kulkarni, S. Boddul, et al. "A chondroprotective potential of root extracts of Withania somnifera in osteoarthritis." *Journal of Bioscience* 32, no. 2 (2007): 299–307.

283. Tandon, N. and S. S. Yadav. "Safety and clinical effectiveness of Withania somnifera (Linn.) dunal root in human ailments." *Journal of Ethnopharmacology* 255 (2020): 112768. doi:10.1016/j.jep.2020.112768

284. Teixeira, M. Y. P. and C. O. Duarte de Araujo. "Effect of Withania somnifera in the treatment of male infertility: A literature review." *Journal of Medicinal Plants Research* 13, no. 8 (2019): 473–479.

285. Tetali, S. D., S. Acharya, A. B. Ankari, et al. "Metabolomics of Withania somnifera (L.) dunal: Advances and applications." *Journal of Ethnopharmacology* 267 (2021): 113469.

286. Thakur, R. S., H. S. Puri and A. Husain. *Major Medicinal Plants of India*, Lucknow, India: CIMAP (1989): 531.

287. Tiwari, R., S. Chakraborty, M. Saminathan, K. Dhama and S. V. Singh. "Ashwagandha (Withania somnifera): Role in safeguarding health, immunomodulatory effects, combating infections, and therapeutic applications: A review." *Journal of Biological Sciences* 14, no. 2 (2014): 77–94.

288. Tohda, C., T. Kuboyama and K. Komatsu. "Search for natural products related to regeneration of the neuronal network." *Neurosignals* 14, no. 2 (2005): 34–45.

289. Tomar, V., T. Beuerle and D. Sircar. "A validated HPTLC method for the simultaneous quantifications of three phenolic acids and three withanolides from Withania somnifera plants and its herbal products." *Journal of Chromatography B* 1124, (2019) 154–160.

290. Trivedi, M. K., P. Panda, K. K. Sethi and S. Jana. "Metabolite profiling of Withania somnifera roots hydroalcoholic extract using LC-MS, GC-MS and NMR spectroscopy." *Chemistry and Biodiversity* 14, no. 3 (2017): e1600280. doi:10.1002/cbdv 201600280

291. Tropicos.org.Missouri Botanical Garden. Accessed 06 July 2021 <https:/tropicos.org/withania somnifera/29600341>

292. Tuli, R. and R. S. Sangwan. *Ashwagandha (Withania Somnifera): A Model Indian Medicinal Plant,* 1st Ed., New Delhi: CSIR-National Botanical Research Institute (2009).

293. Udayakumar, R., S. Kasthurirengan, T. S. Mariashibu, et al. "Hypoglycaemic and hypolipidaemic effects of Withania somnifera root and leaf extracts on alloxan-induced diabetic rats." *International Journal of Molecular Sciences* 10, no. 5(2009): 2367–2382.

294. Uddin, Q., L. Samiulla, V. K. Singh and S. S. Jamil. "Phytochemical and pharmacological profile of Withania somnifera Dunal: A review." *Journal of Applied Pharmaceutical Science* 2, no. 1 (2012): 170–175.

295. Umadevi, M., R. Rajeswari, C. R. Rahale, et al. "Traditional and medicinal uses of Withania somnifera." *The Pharma Innovation* 1, no. 9 (2012): 102–110.

296. Vaishnavi, S., R. Vishwakarma, R. S. Dhar, et al. "Dynamics of withanolide biosynthesis in relation to temporal expression pattern of metabolic genes in Withania somnifera (L.) Dunal: A comparative study in two morpho-chemovariants." *Molecular Biology Reports* 40, no. 12 (2013): 7007–7016.

297. Vareed, S., A. K. Bauer, K. M. Nair, Y. Liu, B. Jayaprakasam and M. G. Nair. "Blood-brain barrier permeability of bioactive withanamides present in Withania somnifera fruit extract." *Phytotherapy Research* 28, no. 8 (2014): 1260–1264.

298. Vedi, M., M. Rasool and E. P. Sabina. "Protective effect of administration of Withania somnifera against bromobenzene induced nephrotoxicity and mitochondrial oxidative stress in rats." *Renal Failure* 36, no. 7 (2014): 1095–1103.

299. Venkataraghavan, S., C. Seshadri, T. P. Sundaresan, et al. "The comparative effect of milk fortified with Ashwagandha, aswagandha and punarnava in children—A double-blind study." *Journal of Research in Ayurveda and Siddha* 1, no. 3 (1980): 370–385.

300. Visavadiya, N. P. and A. V. Narasimhacharya. "Hypocholesteremic and antioxidant effects of Withania somnifera (Dunal) in hypercholesteremic rats." *Phytomedicine* 14, no. 2–3 (2007): 136–142.

301. Vyas, V. K., P. Bhandari and R. Patidar. "A comprehensive review on Withania somnifera Dunal." *Journal of Natural Remedies* 11, no. 1 (2011): 1–13.

302. Wang, F., J. Zhao, J. Bai, et al. "Liquid chromatography-tandem mass spectrometry to assess the pharmacokinetics and tissue distribution of withaferin A in rats." *Journal of Chromatography B Analytical Technologies in the Biomedical and Life Sciences* 1122–1123 (2019): 90–95.

303. Wankhede, S., D. Langade, K. Joshi, S. R. Sinha and S. Bhattacharyya. "Examining the effect of Withania somnifera supplementation on muscle strength and recovery: A randomized controlled trial." *Journal of the International Society of Sports and Nutrition* 12 (2015): 43. doi: 10.1186/s12970-015-0104-9

304. Warrier, P. K., V. P. K. Nambiar and C. Ramankutty. *Indian Medicinal Plants: A Compendium of 500 Species*, Vol. 1, Madras, India: Orient Longman (1996).

305. White, P. T., C. Subramanian, H. F. Motiwala and M. S. Cohen. "Natural withanolides in the treatment of chronic diseases." In S. C. Gupta, S. Prasad and B. B. Aggarwal (eds.) *Anti-Inflammatory Nutraceuticals and Chronic Diseases*, Cham, Switzerland: Springer (2016): 329–373.

306. Winters, M. "Ancient medicine, modern use: Withania somnifera and its potential role in integrative oncology." *Alternative Medicine Review* 11, no. 4 (2006): 269–277.

307. Witter, S., G. Arju, M. Junusova, et al. "Compound's pre-screening of Withania somnifera, bacopa monnieri and Centella asiatica extracts." *Journal of Biosciences and Medicines* 8 (2020): 80–98.

308. Xu, Q.-Q. and K.-W. Wang. "Natural bioactive new withanolides." *Mini Reviews in Medicinal Chemistry* 20, no. 12 (2020): 1101–1117.

309. Zahiruddin S., P. Basist, A. Parveen, et al. Ashwagandha in brain disorders: A review of recent developments. *Journal of Ethnopharmacology* 257 (2020): 112876.

310. Zhang, H. and B. N. Timmermann. "Phytochemical compendium of Withania somnifera (Solanaceae): 1965–2014." *Current Topics in Phytochemistry* 12, (2014): 41–68.

311. Zhao, J., N. Nakamura, M. Hattori, T. Kuboyama, C. Tohda and K. Komatsu. "Withanolide derivatives from the roots of Withania somnifera and their neurite outgrowth activities." *Chemical and Pharmaceutical Bulletin (Tokyo)* 50, no. 6 (2002): 760–765.

Index